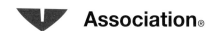 Association®

Pediatric Emergency Assessment, Recognition, and Stabilization

PROVIDER MANUAL

Editors

Leon Chameides, MD, *Content Consultant*

Ricardo A. Samson, MD, *Associate Science Editor*

Stephen M. Schexnayder, MD, *Associate Science Editor*

Mary Fran Hazinski, RN, MSN, *Senior Science Editor*

Senior Managing Editor

Jennifer Ashcraft, RN, BSN

Special Contributors

Marc D. Berg, MD

Allan R. de Caen, MD

Cheryl K. Gooden, MD

Kelly Kadlec, MD

Sharon E. Mace, MD

Brenda Schoolfield, *PEARS Writer*

Mark A. Terry, MPA, NREMT-P

Cindy Tuttle, RN, BSN

Pediatric Subcommittee 2011-2012

Allan R. de Caen, MD, *Chair*

Marc D. Berg, MD, *Immediate Past Chair, 2009-2011*

Dianne L. Atkins, MD

Jeffrey M. Berman, MD

Kathleen Brown, MD

Adam Cheng, MD

Aaron Donoghue, MD, MSCE

Ericka L. Fink, MD

Eugene B. Freid, MD

Cheryl K. Gooden, MD

Melinda L. Fiedor Hamilton, MD, MSc

Kelly Kadlec, MD

Sharon E. Mace, MD

Bradley S. Marino, MD, MPP, MSCE

Craig A. Mathis, MSN, FNP-BC, RNFA

Mary Ann McNeil, MA, NREMT-P

Reylon Meeks, RN, BSN, MS, MSN, EMT, PhD

Vinay Nadkarni, MD

Jeffrey Perlman, MB, ChB

Kennith Hans Sartorelli, MD

© 2012 American Heart Association

ISBN 978-1-61669-247-6

Printed in the United States of America

First American Heart Association Printing June 2012

5 4 3 2

Halden Scott, MD

Wendy Simon, MA

Mark A. Terry, MPA, NREMT-P

Alexis Topjian, MD

Elise W. van der Jagt, MD, MPH

Pediatric Subcommittee 2010-2011

Marc D. Berg, MD, *Chair*

Monica E. Kleinman, MD, *Immediate Past Chair, 2007-2009*

Dianne L. Atkins, MD

Kathleen Brown, MD

Adam Cheng, MD

Laura Conley, BS, RRT, RCP, NPS

Allan R. de Caen, MD

Aaron Donoghue, MD, MSCE

Melinda L. Fiedor Hamilton, MD, MSc

Ericka L. Fink, MD

Eugene B. Freid, MD

Cheryl K. Gooden, MD

Kelly Kadlec, MD

Sharon E. Mace, MD

Bradley S. Marino, MD, MPP, MSCE

Reylon Meeks, RN, BSN, MS, MSN, EMT, PhD

Jeffrey M. Perlman, MB, ChB

Lester Proctor, MD

Faiqa A. Qureshi, MD

Kennith Hans Sartorelli, MD

Wendy Simon, MA

Mark A. Terry, MPA, NREMT-P

Alexis Topjian, MD

Elise W. van der Jagt, MD, MPH

American Academy of Pediatrics Reviewer

Susan Fuchs, MD

Acknowledgment

Special thanks to Edward J. Truemper, MD, for providing the photographs of purpura included in the PEARS DVD.

To find out about any updates or corrections to this text, visit **www.heart.org/cpr**, navigate to the page for this course, and click on "Updates."

Contents

Contents

Preface

The Pediatric Emergency Assessment, Recognition, and Stabilization (PEARS®) Course was developed to better meet the training needs of providers who do not routinely resuscitate infants and children. Although basic life support (BLS) skills are essential for all healthcare providers, not every provider who cares for children applies all of the skills taught in a Pediatric Advanced Life Support (PALS) Course. Specifically, many providers must recognize a child with a potentially life-threatening condition and enlist the help of more advanced providers. Because the recognition of such children is paramount to improving outcomes, this course focuses on improving pediatric assessment and recognition skills, with less emphasis on management.

The initial PEARS Course was the product of work with medical students at the University of Arkansas College of Medicine. This course has been further evaluated and modified to better meet the needs of multiple audiences, including out-of-hospital healthcare providers, in-hospital providers outside of critical care areas, outpatient clinic staff, and school-based providers.

To teach these assessment concepts, the course relies heavily on actual video of real patients with acute conditions. In all cases, consent from the families and/or the patients was obtained, and these patients were receiving high-level acute care in major pediatric medical centers. Importantly, treatment was never delayed to obtain these educational videos. We are grateful to the many families who permitted videotaping to help better educate healthcare professionals in pediatric emergency care. Their generosity in sharing these images will undoubtedly help save the lives of children throughout the world.

Many dedicated volunteers and staff in the Emergency Cardiovascular Care Programs of the American Heart Association have invested thousands of hours in the development and refinement of this course. We hope that these efforts improve the care for ill and injured children by better meeting the educational needs of those who care for these most vulnerable patients.

Stephen M. Schexnayder, MD
Associate Science Editor
American Heart Association, Emergency Cardiovascular Care Programs

General Concepts

Introduction

Course Objectives

Welcome to the Pediatric Emergency Assessment Recognition and Stabilization (PEARS®) Provider Course. It is our hope that as a result of taking this course you will be able to

- Recognize a seriously ill or injured child by using a systematic approach
- Demonstrate high-quality cardiopulmonary resuscitation (CPR)
- Begin to stabilize a seriously ill or injured child
- Practice effective team interaction

Improving Outcome

The earlier you identify severe respiratory distress or shock and start appropriate interventions, the better the chance a seriously ill or injured child has for a good outcome. Once a child is in cardiac arrest, even with optimal resuscitation efforts, outcome is generally poor. According to the *2010 AHA Guidelines for CPR and ECC,* only 4% to 13% of children who have a cardiac arrest in the out-of-hospital setting survive to hospital discharge. The outcome is somewhat better for children in the in-hospital setting: about 27% survive to hospital discharge.

> *Your timely intervention may save the life of a child. If you recognize respiratory distress or shock and intervene quickly, you may prevent progression to cardiac arrest.*

Course Description

To help you achieve the objectives of the PEARS Provider Course, you will participate in the following activities:

- Basic life support (BLS) competency testing
- Rescue breathing skills practice
- Core case discussions
- Cardiac arrest core case simulations
- A video-based written exam

BLS Competency Testing

What You Will Be Expected to Do

You must pass 2 BLS tests to receive an American Heart Association (AHA) PEARS Provider course completion card.

BLS Skills Testing Requirements
• Pass 1- and 2-Rescuer Child BLS With AED Skills Test
• Pass 1- and 2-Rescuer Infant BLS Skills Test

How to Prepare

The PEARS Provider Course does not include detailed instruction about how to perform basic CPR or how to use an automated external defibrillator (AED). You must know this in advance. Consider taking a BLS for Healthcare Providers Course if necessary.

Review the following resources in the *PEARS Provider Manual* to prepare for taking the BLS tests:

Resource	See
BLS skills testing sheets	Part 10: "BLS Competency Testing"
Table 2. Summary of Key BLS Components for Adults, Children, and Infants	Part 12: "Identification and Management of Cardiac Arrest"
Pediatric BLS for Healthcare Providers Algorithm	Part 12: "Identification and Management of Cardiac Arrest" PEARS Pocket Reference Card

Rescue Breathing Skills Practice

What You Will Be Expected to Do

Rescue breathing is a critical skill for PEARS providers. You must be able to provide effective breaths by using a bag-mask device. You should also know when and how to use an oropharyngeal airway (OPA). During the course you will have an opportunity to practice bag-mask ventilation.

How to Prepare

Review the following topics in the *PEARS Provider Manual* to learn more about rescue breathing with a bag and mask (bag-mask ventilation) and an OPA:

Topic	See
Rescue breathing (bag-mask ventilation)	"Rescue Breathing" section in Part 5: "Management of Respiratory Problems"
Bag-mask ventilation	"Equipment and Procedures for Management of Respiratory Emergencies" section in Part 5: "Management of Respiratory Problems"
OPA	

Core Case Discussions

What You Will Be Expected to Do

During the PEARS Course you will watch short video clips of critically ill or injured children. The instructor will lead group discussions, applying the "evaluate-identify-intervene" sequence to each case. Each student is expected to actively participate.

How to Prepare

The focus of the PEARS Course is to teach you to use a systematic approach when caring for a critically ill or injured child. You will need to read and study the entire *PEARS Provider Manual* to understand all the necessary concepts. Targeted resources include the following:

Resource	See
PEARS Systematic Approach Algorithm	Part 2: "PEARS Systematic Approach to the Seriously Ill or Injured Child" PEARS Pocket Reference Card
PEARS Systematic Approach Summary	Appendix PEARS Pocket Reference Card
Management of Respiratory Emergencies Flowchart	
Management of Shock Flowchart	
Vital Signs in Children	
Discussion format for respiratory case discussions	Part 6: "Respiratory Case Discussions"
Discussion format for shock case discussions	Part 9: "Shock Case Discussions"
Discussion format for Putting It All Together case discussions	Part 13: "Putting It All Together Case Discussions"

Cardiac Arrest Core Case Simulations

What You Will Be Expected to Do

During the PEARS Course you will participate as a team member in 2 simulated cardiac arrest cases. You will be expected to perform high-quality CPR and other team roles as directed by your instructor. Your instructor will be the team leader. You also will need to demonstrate good communication skills as outlined in the 8 elements of effective team dynamics.

How to Prepare	Review the following topics in the *PEARS Provider Manual* to prepare yourself to participate as a team member in the cardiac arrest core case simulations:

Topic	See
Team roles and responsibilities	Part 11: "Effective Team Dynamics"
Eight elements of effective team dynamics	
Management of cardiac arrest	Part 12: "Identification and Management of Cardiac Arrest"

Video-Based Written Exam

What You Will Be Expected to Do	The exam is video based. You will receive a handout of written exam questions. The instructor will show a short video clip of a seriously ill or injured child. The video may include vital signs on the screen. The instructor may provide additional information about the case. You will read the test questions related to the clip and write down your answers. There will be several test questions for each clip. You will be allowed to use the PEARS Pocket Reference Card. You may not use the *PEARS Provider Manual*; you may not discuss the cases with another student.
How to Prepare	Prepare *before the class* by reading and studying the *PEARS Provider Manual*. Locate your PEARS Pocket Reference Card and become familiar with the resources available for your reference, such as "Identifying Respiratory Problems" and the Management of Respiratory Emergencies Flowchart. See the "Course Materials" section below for more information about the PEARS Pocket Reference Card.
	Prepare *during the class* by actively participating in the instructor-led core case discussions. Follow along during each case discussion by using the appropriate discussion format in your manual as a guide to learning the systematic approach:

Resource	See
Discussion format for respiratory case discussions	Part 6: "Respiratory Case Discussions"
Discussion format for shock case discussions	Part 9: "Shock Case Discussions"
Discussion format for Putting It All Together case discussions	Part 13: "Putting It All Together Case Discussions"

Course Materials

The PEARS Course materials include the

- *PEARS Provider Manual*
- PEARS Pocket Reference Card

PEARS Provider Manual

The *PEARS Provider Manual* contains material that you will use *before, during,* and *after* the course.

Use the Manual	How
Before the course	Read the entire manual to make sure you have the knowledge you need to participate in the course and pass the video-based written exam. See "What You Will Be Expected to Know" below.
During the course	Use as a reference during • Rescue breathing skills practice • Explanations and demonstrations of equipment • Case discussions
After the course	Refer to specific sections as needed

The manual contains important information that you need to know to effectively participate in the course. ***Please read and study this manual before you come to the course.*** Be sure to take your *PEARS Provider Manual* with you to the course.

PEARS Pocket Reference Card

The PEARS Pocket Reference Card is a valuable learning aid and contains the following resources:

- Vital Signs in Children
- PEARS Systematic Approach Summary
- PEARS Systematic Approach Algorithm
- Identifying Respiratory Problems
- Management of Respiratory Emergencies Flowchart
- Identifying Circulatory Emergencies (Shock)
- Management of Shock Flowchart
- Pediatric BLS for Healthcare Providers Algorithm

Locate the PEARS Systematic Approach Summary and use it to follow along as you read the *PEARS Provider Manual*. Be sure to take your PEARS Pocket Reference Card with you to the course. You will use it as a reference during the core case discussions and the video-based written exam.

What You Will Be Expected to Know

The PEARS Course emphasizes a systematic approach to caring for a seriously ill or injured child (or infant). This approach is designed to help you

- *Evaluate* the child by gathering information about the child's condition
- *Identify* a respiratory problem, a circulatory problem, or both
- *Intervene* with lifesaving actions to treat the problem

This evaluate-identify-intervene approach is discussed in detail in Part 3 of this manual and is shown on the PEARS Pocket Reference Card. You must understand the components of this approach and be able to apply your knowledge during the case discussions. You will demonstrate your understanding of the PEARS Systematic Approach at the end of the course by successfully passing the video-based written exam.

How to Prepare

Read and study the manual to prepare for the course. The manual is organized into the following parts:

	Part	Read to Learn More About...
1	General Concepts	How to prepare to successfully participate in the course and pass the video-based exam
2	PEARS Systematic Approach to the Seriously Ill or Injured Child	An overview of the PEARS Systematic Approach Algorithm
3	Initial Impression and Response	Details about the initial impression; steps to take for an unresponsive child (left side of algorithm) and a responsive child (right side of algorithm)
4	Airway and Breathing: Primary Assessment and Identification of Respiratory Problems	The A and B components of the primary assessment; how to identify the 4 types of respiratory problems
5	Management of Respiratory Problems	Initial interventions for a child with a respiratory problem; specific interventions based on identification of the problem
6	Respiratory Case Discussions	Discussion format for instructor-led group discussions of the systematic approach to a child with a respiratory problem
7	Circulation, Disability, and Exposure: Primary Assessment and Identification of Shock	The C, D, and E components of the primary assessment; how to identify hypovolemic and distributive shock
8	Management of Circulatory Emergencies (Shock)	Initial interventions for a child in shock
9	Shock Case Discussions	Discussion format for instructor-led group discussions of the systematic approach to a child in shock
10	BLS Competency Testing	The criteria that your instructor will use to test you on your BLS skills
11	Effective Team Dynamics	The 8 elements of effective team dynamics; summary of team roles and responsibilities
12	Identification and Management of Cardiac Arrest	Signs of cardiac arrest; basic life support
13	Putting It All Together Case Discussions	Discussion format for instructor-led group discussions of the PEARS Systematic Approach to a child with a respiratory or circulatory problem

(continued)

(continued)

Part	Read to Learn More About...
Appendix	Valuable tools to use before, during, and after the course, including Vital Signs in Children, PEARS Systematic Approach Algorithm, PEARS Systematic Approach Summary, Management of Respiratory Emergencies Flowchart, Management of Shock Flowchart

Detailed and Advanced Concepts	The green call-out boxes throughout this manual are used to present more detailed or advanced concepts. Much of this content was developed by the AHA Subcommittee on Pediatric Resuscitation. The information is based on years of experience and research in the field of pediatric advanced life support.

Course Completion Requirements

To successfully complete the PEARS Provider Course and obtain your course completion card, you must do the following:

- Actively participate in the case discussions
- Actively participate in the Rescue Breathing Skills Station and cardiac arrest case simulations
- Pass the skills tests in 1- and 2-rescuer child BLS with AED and 1- and 2-rescuer infant BLS
- Pass the video-based written exam with a minimum score of 84%

Science Update

The PEARS Provider Course has been updated to reflect new science changes. Every few years hundreds of international resuscitation scientists and experts evaluate, discuss, and debate thousands of scientific publications. They reach consensus on the best treatments based on the evidence that they have evaluated. These consensus recommendations form the basis for the development of the guidelines. *The 2010 AHA Guidelines for CPR and ECC* is based on the largest review of resuscitation literature ever published. Some recommendations are new, whereas others modify previous recommendations.

Major Science Changes in 2010

Some of the major science changes in 2010 include

- Recommendation for immediate chest compressions for a child who is unresponsive and not breathing or only gasping (C-A-B vs A-B-C)
- Continued emphasis on high-quality CPR, including minor changes to depth of compressions
- Recommendations about the use of an AED for infants

It is hoped that these changes will result in more lives saved.

Immediate Chest Compressions (C-A-B vs A-B-C)

The *2010 AHA Guidelines for CPR and ECC* recommended a change in the CPR sequence from A-B-C (Airway-Breathing-Circulation/Compressions) to C-A-B (Compressions-Airway-Breathing). The change to C-A-B was made for the following reasons:

- Only about 30% of victims of sudden death receive any bystander CPR. One of the obstacles to bystander CPR may be the difficulty in opening the airway and giving ventilation. Chest compressions are more easily taught and performed. This may help increase performance of bystander CPR.
- Compressions require no equipment, so CPR can be started immediately without delay.
- The vast majority of cardiac arrest victims are adults with sudden cardiac arrest. Sudden cardiac arrest is best treated with immediate chest compressions and defibrillation.
- Although a combination of chest compressions and ventilation is required for pediatric arrest, the C-A-B sequence should delay the start of ventilation by about 18 seconds or less for a single rescuer and 9 seconds or less for 2 rescuers.
- A uniform C-A-B sequence for victims of all ages (excluding newly born infants) should be easy to learn, remember, and perform.

Emphasis on High-Quality CPR

High-quality CPR is essential. Without the foundation of effective BLS, even the most advanced life support measures will fail.

High-quality CPR is critical during cardiac arrest to provide adequate blood flow to the brain and vital organs. Compressions generate blood flow. Every time compressions are interrupted, blood flow stops. When chest compressions are resumed, it takes several compressions before blood flow reaches the level it was before the interruption.

Critical elements of high-quality CPR include the following:

Push fast	• Push at a rate of at least 100 compressions per minute.
Push hard	• Push with enough force to depress the chest at least one third the depth of the chest. This is about 1.5 inches (4 cm) in infants and 2 inches (5 cm) in children.
Allow full chest recoil	• *Release completely,* allowing the chest to fully recoil after each compression. This allows the heart to refill with blood.
Minimize interruptions	• Try to limit interruptions in chest compressions to 10 seconds or less or as needed for interventions (eg, defibrillation). Ideally, compressions are interrupted only for ventilation (until an advanced airway is placed), rhythm check, and actual shock delivery. • Once an advanced airway is in place, provide continuous chest compressions without pausing for ventilation.
Avoid excessive ventilation	• Each rescue breath should take about 1 second. Each breath should result in visible chest rise. • After an advanced airway is in place, deliver 8 to 10 breaths/min (1 breath every 6 to 8 seconds), being careful to avoid excessive ventilation.

Use of AEDs in Infants

If a victim of cardiac arrest has a shockable rhythm, survival requires CPR and defibrillation. For an infant, use a manual defibrillator, if possible, instead of an AED.

If a manual defibrillator is not available or there is no one present trained to use one, use an AED. An AED capable of giving a pediatric dose is preferred for use in infants and in children younger than 8 years. If neither is available, an AED without a pediatric dose setting may be used. For an infant in cardiac arrest with a shockable rhythm, a high-dose shock is better than no shock.

References

For further reading and study and for detailed references, see the following publications:

2010 American Heart Association Guidelines for Cardiopulmonary Resuscitation and Emergency Cardiovascular Care. *Circulation.* 2010;122(suppl 3):S639-S946. www.heart.org/eccguidelines. Accessed January 3, 2012.

2010 Handbook of Emergency Cardiovascular Care for Healthcare Providers. Dallas, TX: American Heart Association; 2010.

American Heart Association. 2010 International Consensus on Cardiopulmonary Resuscitation and Emergency Cardiovascular Care Science With Treatment Recommendations. *Circulation.* 2010;122(suppl 2):S249-S638.

American Heart Association. *Highlights of the 2010 American Heart Association Guidelines for CPR and ECC.* Dallas, TX: American Heart Association; 2010. www.heart.org/eccguidelines. Accessed January 3, 2012.

Pediatric Advanced Life Support Provider Manual. Dallas, TX: American Heart Association; 2011.

Part 2

PEARS Systematic Approach to the Seriously Ill or Injured Child

Overview

A PEARS provider should use a systematic approach when caring for a seriously ill or injured child. The purpose of this organized approach is to help you quickly identify a child at risk for cardiac arrest and provide lifesaving interventions.

Learning Objectives

After completing this Part you should be able to

- Define the initial impression
- Explain when to use the left side of the PEARS Systematic Approach Algorithm
- Explain when to use the right side of the PEARS Systematic Approach Algorithm

Preparation for the Course

During the course you will actively participate in case discussions after watching short videos of critically ill or injured pediatric patients. Your answers will be guided by the PEARS Systematic Approach Algorithm, including the evaluate-identify-intervene sequence. Locate this algorithm in the Appendix for future reference.

PEARS Systematic Approach Algorithm

The PEARS Systematic Approach Algorithm (Figure 1) outlines the approach to caring for a critically ill or injured child.

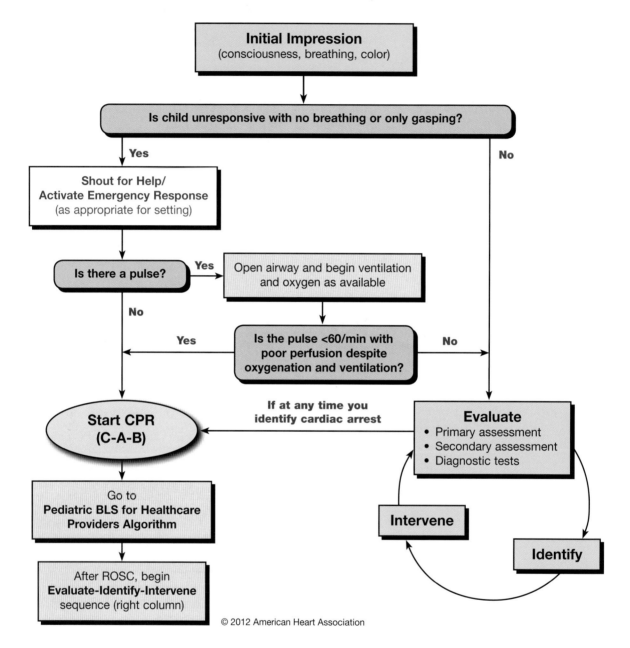

© 2012 American Heart Association

Figure 1. PEARS Systematic Approach Algorithm.

If at any time you identify a life-threatening problem, immediately begin appropriate interventions. Activate emergency response as indicated in your practice setting.

Identify a Life-Threatening Condition

The initial impression (Figure 1) is your first quick "from the doorway" observation. It is accomplished within the *first few seconds* of encountering the child. The purpose of this assessment is to quickly identify a life-threatening condition.

If the child's condition is...	Then the next action is to...
Life threatening	• Start life support interventions • Get help
Not life threatening	• Continue with the systematic approach

During the initial impression, look and listen to gather information about

- Consciousness
- Breathing
- Color

See Part 3 for more information on how to evaluate consciousness, breathing, and color.

Child Unresponsive and Not Breathing or Only Gasping

Follow Left Side of Algorithm

If the child is **unresponsive** and not breathing or only gasping, follow the left side of the algorithm. Call for help and provide CPR or rescue breathing as needed.

Child Responsive and Breathing

Follow Right Side of Algorithm

If the child is **responsive** and breathing, continue with the right side of the algorithm. You will *evaluate* the child by using the ABCDE components of the primary assessment:

A	Airway
B	Breathing
C	Circulation
D	Disability
E	Exposure

For more information on airway and breathing, see Part 4. From more information on circulation, disability, and exposure, see Part 7. The information from your evaluation will help you to *identify* the problem and *intervene* with appropriate treatment.

Part 3

Initial Impression and Response

Overview

Rapid intervention may be lifesaving for a critically ill or injured child. If a child is unresponsive with no breathing or only gasping, the child needs CPR. If the child is not breathing but has a pulse, the child needs rescue breathing. You should provide CPR or rescue breathing as needed and get help. There is no time to waste trying to make decisions about what to do. Learning the concepts presented in the PEARS Systematic Approach Algorithm will give you the knowledge you need to respond quickly to a pediatric emergency.

Note: Providers should be aware of potential environmental dangers when providing care. In out-of-hospital settings, always assess the scene before you evaluate the child.

Learning Objectives

After completing this Part you should be able to

- Explain the steps to take if a child is unresponsive with no breathing or only gasping
- List and define the components of the initial impression
- Discuss the evaluate-identify-intervene sequence

Preparation for the Course

The PEARS Systematic Approach Algorithm is a fundamental concept of the PEARS Course. You must understand the steps in the algorithm to be successful in the course.

Begin Initial Impression

As you learned in Part 2, the initial impression is your first quick "from the doorway" observation. It is accomplished within the *first few seconds* of encountering the child. During the initial impression, look and listen to gather information about

- Consciousness
- Breathing
- Color

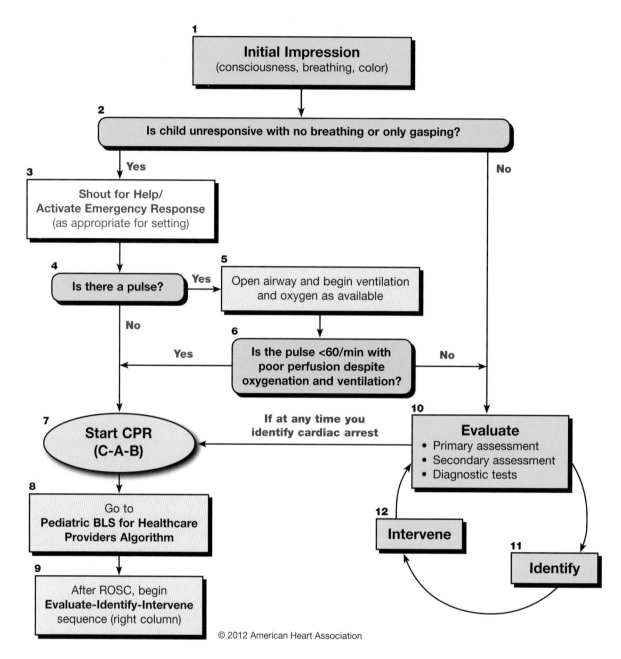

Figure 1. PEARS Systematic Approach Algorithm.

The algorithm boxes contain the following text:

1. **Initial Impression** (consciousness, breathing, color)

2. **Is child unresponsive with no breathing or only gasping?**
   - Yes → (box 3)
   - No → (box 10 Evaluate)

3. **Shout for Help/ Activate Emergency Response** (as appropriate for setting)

4. **Is there a pulse?**
   - Yes → (box 5)
   - No → (box 7)

5. Open airway and begin ventilation and oxygen as available

6. **Is the pulse <60/min with poor perfusion despite oxygenation and ventilation?**
   - Yes → (box 7)
   - No → (box 10 Evaluate)

7. **Start CPR (C-A-B)**

If at any time you identify cardiac arrest

8. Go to **Pediatric BLS for Healthcare Providers Algorithm**

9. After ROSC, begin **Evaluate-Identify-Intervene** sequence (right column)

10. **Evaluate**
    - Primary assessment
    - Secondary assessment
    - Diagnostic tests

11. **Identify**

12. **Intervene**

© 2012 American Heart Association

Consciousness

Carefully, but quickly, observe the child's appearance to evaluate the level of consciousness. Is it normal or abnormal? Is the child unresponsive, less responsive, or irritable? Is the child alert?

If the child is crying or upset, it can be difficult to know if the child is responding appropriately. Try to keep the child as calm as possible. Let her remain with her parent or caregiver if practical. Use distractions such as toys.

Breathing

During the initial impression, you evaluate the child's breathing *without a stethoscope*. (Later during the primary assessment you will use a stethoscope.) Look for signs of absent, increased, or inadequate respiratory effort. Listen for sounds of abnormal breathing. Observe the respiratory rate. During the initial impression you may identify signs of mild respiratory distress, severe respiratory distress, or respiratory arrest. Assess respiratory effort and lung and airway sounds. *Is the breathing normal or abnormal?*

	Normal	**Abnormal**
Respiratory effort*	• Regular breathing, no increased effort • Passive expiration	• Nasal flaring • Retractions or use of abdominal muscles • Increased, inadequate, or absent respiratory effort
Lung and airway sounds*	No abnormal respiratory sounds audible	Noisy breathing (eg, wheezing, grunting, or stridor)

*See the detailed discussion of respiratory effort and lung and airway sounds in the section on primary assessment in Part 4.

Color

Evaluate the child's color. You can often identify important information about circulatory status just by looking at a child. When the amount of blood pumped by the heart (cardiac output) is too low, the body reduces circulation to nonessential areas, such as the skin and mucous membranes. This is an attempt to preserve blood supply to the brain and heart. Therefore, skin color and overall skin appearance provide important clues to help identify circulatory problems.

Pallor (paleness), mottling (an irregular skin color), and cyanosis (bluish color) may be signs of inadequate cardiac output. Cyanosis of the lips and fingernails may be present if the child is unable to adequately oxygenate the blood.

Observe the exposed parts of the child, such as the face, arms, and legs. Inspection of the skin may reveal bruising that suggests injury. You may also see evidence of bleeding within the skin, called petechiae or purpura. This purplish discoloration of the skin is often a sign of a life-threatening infection.

Evaluate the skin and mucous membranes. *Are they normal or abnormal?*

	Normal	**Abnormal**
Skin color*	Appears normal	• Pallor • Mottling • Cyanosis
Hemorrhage	No obvious bleeding	• Obvious significant bleeding • Bleeding within the skin (eg, purpura)

*See the discussion of skin color in the section on primary assessment in Part 4.

Unresponsive or Responsive

The purpose of the initial impression is to quickly identify a life-threatening condition.

If...	Then...
The child is unresponsive	Immediately determine if lifesaving intervention is needed (ie, if cardiac or respiratory arrest is present). If the child is unresponsive with no breathing or only gasping, shout for help. Provide CPR or rescue breathing as needed.
The child is responsive and breathing	Continue with the evaluate-identify-intervene sequence.

If Child Is Unresponsive in Respiratory or Cardiac Arrest

If Child Is Unresponsive

During the initial impression you evaluate the child's consciousness, breathing, and color to quickly identify a life-threatening condition. If the child is unresponsive with no breathing or only gasping, you will proceed down the left side of the PEARS Systematic Approach Algorithm (Figure 1). In the text that follows, box numbers refer to the corresponding boxes in this algorithm.

Activate Emergency Response (Box 2)

If the child is unresponsive and not breathing or only gasping (Box 2), shout for help or activate emergency response as appropriate for your practice setting (Box 3).

Pulse Check (Box 4)

Check for a pulse (Box 4).

No Pulse

If there is no pulse, start CPR, beginning with chest compressions (Box 7). Proceed according to the Pediatric BLS for Healthcare Providers Algorithm. After return of spontaneous circulation (ROSC), begin the evaluate-identify-intervene sequence (Boxes 10-12).

A Pulse Is Present

If a pulse is present, open the airway and provide rescue breathing (Box 5). Use oxygen as soon as it is available. See "Rescue Breathing" in Part 5 for more information. For infants and children, give 1 breath every 3 to 5 seconds (about 12 to 20 breaths/min). Give each breath in 1 second. Each breath should result in visible chest rise. Check the heart rate.

If Heart Rate Is	Next Steps
Less than 60/min with signs of poor perfusion despite adequate oxygenation and ventilation (Box 6)	Provide chest compressions and ventilation (Box 7). Proceed according to the Pediatric BLS for Healthcare Providers Algorithm (Box 8).
Greater than 60/min	Continue ventilation as needed. Begin the evaluate-identify-intervene sequence (Boxes 10-12). You should check the pulse about every 2 minutes. If at any time the child demonstrates a life-threatening problem, begin appropriate Intervention (eg, CPR) and call for help.

Breathing Is Adequate	If the child is breathing adequately, proceed with the evaluate-identify-intervene sequence.

> *If at any time you identify a life-threatening problem, immediately begin appropriate interventions. Activate emergency response as indicated in your practice setting.*

Rescue Breathing	During the PEARS Course you will have an opportunity to demonstrate rescue breathing by using a bag-mask device. See Part 5: "Management of Respiratory Problems" for information on rescue breathing and bag-mask ventilation.

If Child Is Responsive

Evaluate-Identify-Intervene Sequence

Evaluate-Identify-Intervene (Boxes 10-12)	If the child is responsive, proceed down the right side of the PEARS Systematic Approach Algorithm (Figure 1). Begin the evaluate-identify-intervene sequence (Boxes 10-12). This will help you determine the best treatment or intervention at any point. From the information gathered during your evaluation (Box 10), identify the child's clinical condition by type and severity (Box 11). Intervene with appropriate actions (Box 12). Then repeat the sequence. This process is ongoing.

> *Always look for a life-threatening problem. If at any time you identify a life-threatening problem, immediately begin appropriate interventions. Activate emergency response as indicated in your practice setting*

Evaluate	If no life-threatening problem is present, evaluation of the child's condition may continue with clinical assessment tools described below.

Clinical Assessment	Brief Description
Primary assessment	A rapid, hands-on ABCDE approach to evaluate respiratory, cardiac, and neurologic function; this step includes assessment of vital signs and pulse oximetry
Secondary assessment	A focused medical history and a focused physical examination
Diagnostic tests	Laboratory, radiographic, and other advanced tests that help identify the child's condition and diagnosis

The *PEARS Provider Manual* discusses the primary assessment in detail. Pediatric advanced life support (PALS) providers usually perform the secondary assessment and order diagnostic tests. Although these terms suggest that one assessment follows the other, several parts of each assessment are usually done at the same time. You should adjust your assessment approach on the basis of the child's clinical condition and history. For more information about secondary assessment and diagnostic tests, see the *PALS Provider Manual*.

Identify

On the basis of your evaluation, try to identify the type and severity of the child's clinical condition.

	Type	Severity
Respiratory	• Upper airway obstruction • Lower airway obstruction • Lung tissue disease • Disordered control of breathing	• Mild respiratory distress • Severe respiratory distress*
Circulatory	• Hypovolemic shock • Distributive shock • Cardiogenic shock† • Obstructive shock†	• Compensated shock • Hypotensive shock

*PEARS providers are not expected to identify a child in respiratory distress versus a child in respiratory failure. This course focuses on early identification of respiratory problems and early intervention.

†The PEARS Provider Course does not cover recognition or treatment of cardiogenic and obstructive shock.

The child's clinical condition can result from a combination of respiratory and circulatory problems. As the condition of a seriously ill or injured child worsens, one problem may lead to others. For example, a child in shock may develop respiratory distress.

> Note that in the initial phase of your identification, you may be uncertain about the type or severity of problems, or both. It is important to reevaluate as you intervene because both the type and severity of problems may change.

Identifying the child's problem is important because it helps you prioritize the best initial interventions.

Intervene

On the basis of your identification of the child's clinical condition, intervene with appropriate actions. Your actions will be determined by your scope of practice and local protocol. Interventions for PEARS providers may include

- Getting help by activating a medical emergency or rapid response team
- Starting CPR
- Obtaining an AED, code cart, or monitor/defibrillator
- Attaching a heart monitor and a pulse oximeter
- Positioning the child
- Giving oxygen
- Providing nebulizer therapy or using an epinephrine autoinjector
- Giving a fluid bolus

The best action may be to get help. Provide emergency support until help arrives. Be prepared to assist as a member of the team after more advanced providers take over the child's care.

Ongoing Sequence

The sequence of evaluate-identify-intervene is ongoing until the child is stable. Remember to repeat the evaluate-identify-intervene sequence

- After each intervention
- When the child's condition changes or deteriorates

Use this sequence to look for trends in the child's condition. For example, after you give oxygen, reevaluate the child. Is the child more responsive (eg, is consciousness improved)? Has the child's respiratory effort changed? Has the child's color improved? After giving a fluid bolus to a child in hypovolemic shock, do the child's heart rate and perfusion improve? Is another bolus needed? Use evaluate-identify-intervene after each intervention and whenever the child's condition changes.

> *If at any time you identify a life-threatening problem, immediately begin appropriate interventions. Activate emergency response as indicated in your practice setting.*

Part 4

Airway and Breathing: Primary Assessment and Identification of Respiratory Problems

Introduction

Use the evaluate-identify-intervene sequence for any seriously ill or injured child. Begin with the primary assessment. This Part gives a brief overview of the primary assessment and then focuses on evaluation of airway (A) and breathing (B). This information will help you identify respiratory problems.

First determine if the child is breathing or not breathing.

If...	Then...
The child is not breathing or only gasping	Start CPR immediately
The child is breathing	Gather information to identify • No distress • Mild respiratory distress • Severe respiratory distress

In infants and children, respiratory problems can quickly progress to severe distress and cardiac arrest. Good outcome (ie, survival to hospital discharge with good neurologic function) is more likely if you intervene early. Once the child is in cardiac arrest, outcome is generally poor.

> *You can greatly improve outcome by early identification and management of respiratory problems.*

Learning Objectives

After completing this Part you should be able to

- Summarize the A and B components of the primary assessment
- List the 5 elements in evaluation of breathing: respiratory rate and pattern, respiratory effort, chest expansion and air movement, lung and airway sounds, and oxygen saturation by pulse oximetry
- Identify signs and symptoms of upper airway obstruction, lower airway obstruction, lung tissue disease, and disordered control of breathing
- Recognize the signs of mild and severe respiratory distress
- Recognize the signs of inadequate oxygenation and inadequate ventilation

Preparation for the Course

A systematic evaluation of airway and breathing is fundamental in the care of any seriously ill or injured child. As you study this chapter, refer to the PEARS Systematic Approach Summary located in the Appendix and on the PEARS Pocket Reference Card.

Primary Assessment Overview

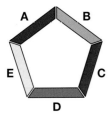

As you recall, the initial impression is your first quick "from the doorway" observation of the child. During the initial impression you use what you see and hear to gather information before you even touch the child. In contrast, the primary assessment is a *hands-on* evaluation. Here you use an ABCDE approach to assess

- **A**irway
- **B**reathing
- **C**irculation
- **D**isability
- **E**xposure

The primary assessment will help you identify the type and severity of the child's problem. This assessment includes evaluation of vital signs and oxygen saturation by pulse oximetry. It also includes a rapid blood glucose test if needed.

> *Important: During each step of the primary assessment, watch for any signs of a life-threatening problem. If at any time you identify a life-threatening problem, immediately begin appropriate interventions. Activate emergency response as indicated in your practice setting.*

Once any life-threatening problems are addressed and the primary assessment is completed, an advanced provider should perform the secondary assessment and order diagnostic tests.

In the *PEARS Provider Manual,* discussion of the primary assessment is divided into 2 parts:

Primary Assessment Components	Discussed in
Airway and **B**reathing	Part 4: "Airway and Breathing: Primary Assessment and Identification of Respiratory Problems"
Circulation, **D**isability, and **E**xposure	Part 7: "Circulation, Disability, and Exposure: Primary Assessment and Identification of Shock"

Primary Assessment: Airway and Breathing

Airway

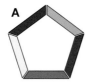

Evaluate Airway	Assess the airway to determine whether it is open and clear or obstructed. Evaluate the following:

- Look for movement of the chest or abdomen
- Listen for bilateral breath sounds and air movement
- Feel for movement of air at the nose and mouth

If there is some airway obstruction, you then decide if the airway is maintainable or not maintainable.

Status	Description
Clear	Airway is open and unobstructed for normal breathing.
Maintainable	Airway is obstructed but can be opened (maintained) by *simple measures,* such as positioning or insertion of an oropharyngeal airway (OPA).
Not maintainable	Airway is obstructed and cannot be maintained without *advanced interventions,* such as intubation.

If you think that the airway is obstructed, you must decide where the obstruction is located. The obstruction may be in the upper airway. Signs that suggest the upper airway is obstructed are

- Increased inspiratory effort with retractions
- Abnormal inspiratory sounds (snoring or high-pitched stridor)
- Decreased air movement despite increased respiratory effort

If the upper airway is obstructed, try to maintain an open airway with *simple measures*. If you cannot maintain the airway with simple measures, get help for *advanced treatment*.

Simple Measures to Maintain the Airway	Simple measures to open the upper airway and maintain patency may include one or more of the following:

Positioning	Allow the child to assume a position of comfort or position the child to open the airway.
	For a responsive child
	• Allow the child to assume a position of comfort *or*
	• Elevate the head of the bed
	For an unresponsive child
	• Turn the child on her side if you do not suspect cervical injury *or*
	• Use a head tilt–chin lift or jaw thrust (below)

(continued)

(continued)

Head tilt–chin lift or jaw thrust	• *If you do not suspect cervical spine injury*: Use a head tilt–chin lift to open the airway. Avoid overextending the head/neck in infants because this may occlude the airway. • *If you suspect cervical spine injury:* Open the airway by using a jaw thrust *without* neck extension. Opening the airway is a priority. If a jaw thrust does not open the airway, use a head tilt–chin lift or a head tilt with a jaw thrust despite a possible cervical spine injury. Note that the jaw thrust also may be used to open the airway in a child without suspected cervical spinal injury.
Suctioning	Suction the nose and oropharynx.
Relief techniques for foreign-body airway obstruction	If a foreign-body airway obstruction (FBAO) is present, relieve the obstruction in a *responsive child* by the following: • If the child is younger than 1 year of age: give 5 back blows (slaps) and 5 chest compressions. • If the child is 1 year of age or older: give abdominal thrusts. If at any time the child becomes unresponsive, begin CPR and send someone to activate emergency response.
Airway adjuncts	Use airway adjuncts (eg, insert an OPA).

Advanced Treatment to Maintain the Airway

The child may need advanced treatment to maintain the airway. Advanced providers perform these interventions, which may include one or more of the following:

- Placing an advanced airway (eg, endotracheal tube)
- Applying continuous positive airway pressure (CPAP) or noninvasive positive-pressure breathing assistance
- Removing a foreign body; this may require looking at the airway with a laryngoscope
- Creating a surgical opening through the skin into the trachea

Breathing

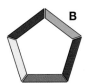

B

Evaluate Breathing

Assess breathing by evaluating

- Respiratory rate and pattern
- Respiratory effort
- Chest expansion and air movement
- Lung and airway sounds
- Oxygen saturation by pulse oximetry

Normal Respiratory Rate and Pattern

Normal breathing takes little work: breathing is quiet, with unlabored inspiration and passive expiration. The child looks comfortable. The normal respiratory rate is typically faster in younger infants and children than in older children (Table 1).

Try to evaluate the respiratory rate before you touch the child. If the child becomes anxious or upset, the respiratory rate will often increase.

To determine the respiratory rate, count the number of times the chest rises in 30 seconds and multiply by 2. Be aware that normal sleeping infants may have irregular breathing with pauses lasting up to 10 or even 15 seconds. If you count chest rises for less than 30 seconds, you may not estimate the rate accurately. Count the respiratory rate several times as you assess and reassess the child to detect changes. Many cardiac monitors also have the ability to continuously monitor the respiratory rate.

Table 1. Normal Respiratory Rates by Age

Age	Breaths/min
Infant (younger than 1 year)	30 to 60
Toddler (1 to 3 years)	24 to 40
Preschooler (4 to 5 years)	22 to 34
School–age child (6 to 12 years)	18 to 30
Adolescent (13 to 18 years)	12 to 16

Reproduced from Hazinski MF. Children are different. In: Hazinski MF. *Manual of Pediatric Critical Care.* St Louis, MO: Mosby; 1999:1-13, copyright Elsevier. From Hazinski MF. Children are different. In: Hazinski MF. *Nursing Care of the Critically Ill Child*. 2nd ed. St Louis, MO: Mosby-Year Book; 1992:1-17, copyright Elsevier.

A consistent respiratory rate of less than 10 breaths/min or more than 60 breaths/min in a child of any age is abnormal. Such a slow or rapid respiratory rate suggests a serious condition and requires immediate intervention.

Detailed and Advanced Concepts

Be careful to consider the child's clinical condition when you evaluate the respiratory rate and pattern.

- An increase in respiratory rate may be appropriate if the child has a fever or if the child is ill or in pain.
- A decrease in respiratory rate from fast to "normal" may indicate overall improvement. Improvement should be accompanied by an increased level of consciousness. The child who is improving should also show decreased work of breathing.
- A decreasing respiratory rate or irregular respiratory pattern may also indicate that the child's clinical condition is worsening. The child's general appearance or signs of circulation will often change as the child's condition worsens. Skin color may become pale, mottled, or cyanotic. The child's level of consciousness may decrease.

Abnormal Respiratory Rate and Pattern

Abnormal respirations include

- Irregular respiratory pattern
- Fast respiratory rate
- Slow respiratory rate
- Apnea

Irregular Respiratory Pattern

Children with neurologic problems may have irregular respiratory patterns. Examples of such irregular patterns are

- A deep gasping breath, followed by a period of breath holding
- A rapid respiratory rate, followed by periods of apnea or very shallow breaths

Irregular patterns such as these are serious and require urgent evaluation.

Fast Respiratory Rate

A *fast respiratory rate* (tachypnea) is a breathing rate that is faster than normal for age. This is often the first sign of respiratory distress in infants. Tachypnea can also develop during periods of stress.

A fast respiratory rate may or may not be accompanied by signs of increased respiratory effort. A fast respiratory rate *without* signs of increased respiratory effort may result from

- Conditions that do not involve the respiratory system, such as high fever, pain, and sepsis (serious infection)
- Dehydration

Slow Respiratory Rate

A slower than normal respiratory rate may be caused by

- Fatigue
- A central nervous system injury or problem that affects the respiratory control center
- Very low blood oxygen concentration (ie, low oxygen saturation, indicated by pulse oximetry or cyanosis)
- Sepsis
- Hypothermia
- Drugs that depress the respiratory drive
- Some muscle diseases that cause muscle weakness

Detailed and Advanced Concepts	A slow respiratory rate or an irregular respiratory rate in a severely ill or injured infant or child is a sign of a serious problem. It often signals that the child may soon develop respiratory arrest. If you encounter such a child, immediately activate emergency response and be prepared to provide rescue breathing.

Apnea

Apnea is a pause in breathing for at least 20 seconds. Apnea is also present if the pause is less than 20 seconds and other signs of inadequate breathing are present. Other signs of inadequate breathing can include slow heart rate, cyanosis, or pallor.

Increased Respiratory Effort

Evaluate respiratory effort to assess the severity of the child's condition and the need for urgent intervention. The following are signs of increased respiratory effort:

- Nasal flaring
- Retractions
- Head bobbing or seesaw respirations

Other signs of increased respiratory effort are prolonged inspiration or expiration and open-mouth breathing. Grunting is a serious sign that may indicate severe respiratory distress. See "Grunting" later in this section.

The child who has increased respiratory effort is trying to improve the level of oxygen in the body (oxygenation) or is trying to improve carbon dioxide elimination (ventilation) or both.

Nasal Flaring

Nasal flaring is a widening of the nostrils during each inspiration. The nostrils open to maximize airflow during breathing. Nasal flaring is most commonly seen in infants and younger children. It is usually a sign of respiratory distress.

Retractions

Retractions are an inward movement of the chest wall, neck, or sternum during inspiration. Retractions may occur in several areas of the chest, as noted in the table below. In more severe cases, retractions may be present in all of these areas.

Retractions are a sign of increased respiratory effort. The child is using chest muscles to try to move air into the lungs. However, air movement is impaired by narrowing of the airways or by stiff lungs. The severity of the retractions generally corresponds to the severity of respiratory distress.

The following table describes the location of retractions commonly seen with each level of breathing difficulty:

Breathing Difficulty	Location of Retractions	Description
Mild to moderate	Subcostal	Retractions of the abdomen, just below the rib cage
	Substernal	Retractions of the abdomen, at the bottom of the breastbone
	Intercostal	Retractions between the ribs
Severe (may also include the same retractions as seen with mild-to-moderate breathing difficulty)	Supraclavicular	Retractions in the neck, just above the collarbone
	Suprasternal	Retractions in the chest, just above the breastbone
	Sternal	Retractions of the sternum towards the spine

Signs that accompany retractions are often clues to the cause of the child's condition, such as the following:

- Retractions that are present with stridor or an inspiratory snoring sound suggest upper airway obstruction.
- Retractions with expiratory wheezing suggest marked lower airway obstruction (asthma or bronchiolitis), causing obstruction during both inspiration and expiration
- Retractions with grunting or labored breathing suggest lung tissue disease

Severe chest retractions may also be accompanied by head bobbing or seesaw respirations.

Head Bobbing or Seesaw Respirations

Head bobbing and seesaw respirations are signs of severe respiratory distress. These signs often suggest that the child's condition may worsen. If you see these signs, you should get help.

- *Head bobbing* is caused by the use of neck muscles to assist breathing. During inspiration the child lifts his chin and extends his neck. During expiration his chin falls forward. Head bobbing is most frequently seen in infants.
- *Seesaw respirations* are a distinct form of "abdominal breathing." During inspiration the chest retracts inward and the abdomen expands. During expiration the chest expands and the abdomen moves inward. Note that normal infants can have abdominal breathing, with the abdomen rising during inspiration. With normal abdominal breathing, no other signs of increased respiratory effort are present.

Inadequate Respiratory Effort

In your evaluation of respiratory effort, look for signs that respiratory effort is inadequate. These include

- Apnea
- Weak cry or cough

Chest Expansion and Air Movement

To assess chest expansion and air movement, you should

- Observe chest wall movement
- Listen for air movement with a stethoscope

Determine if chest expansion and air movement are normal, decreased, or unequal. Also look for prolonged expiration. Prolonged expiration is an increase in the time it takes the child to exhale. It is usually a sign of lower airway obstruction (eg, asthma).

Chest Expansion

Chest expansion (chest rise) during inspiration should be equal (symmetrical) on both sides of the chest. Expansion may be subtle during spontaneous quiet breathing when the chest is covered by clothing. But chest expansion should be easy to see when the chest is uncovered. In normal infants the abdomen may move more than the chest during inspiration. Some causes of decreased or unequal chest expansion are

- Inadequate effort
- Airway obstruction (narrowing of the small airways or presence of secretions in the larger airways)
- Aspiration of a foreign body
- Collapse of all or part of the lungs
- Air, blood, or fluid in the space surrounding the lungs

Air Movement

It is important to listen to air movement as air enters and exits from the lungs. Using a stethoscope, listen to the following areas to determine whether air movement is normal or decreased:

Area	Location
Anterior	Mid chest (just to the left and right of the sternum)
Lateral	Under the armpits (the best location for evaluating air movement into the lower parts of the lungs)
Posterior	Both sides of the back

Compare air movement in one area with sounds heard over other areas. You may hear normal air movement in some parts of the chest but decreased air movement in other areas.

Note the quality of air movement. Because the child's chest wall is thin, it is easy to hear air movement or airway sounds in one part of the chest when your stethoscope is over another part of the chest. You may also hear sounds from the upper airway when you listen all over the chest. This is because sound is easily transmitted through the chest from the upper airway.

Listen to the loudness of the air movement:

- Normal inspiratory sounds should be soft and quiet. Watch the movement of the child's chest as the child inhales. Inspiratory sounds should occur at the same time as the chest movement.
- Normal expiratory breath sounds are often short and even quieter than inspiratory sounds. You may not even hear the sound of normal expiration.

You may have difficulty hearing air movement and airway sounds at all in an obese child. In this case it will be especially difficult to identify abnormalities. Look for signs of distress by assessing the child's respiratory effort.

Lung and Airway Sounds

During the primary assessment you should evaluate the child for abnormal lung and airway sounds. Some abnormal sounds are stridor, snoring, barking cough, and hoarseness. Grunting, gurgling, wheezing, and crackles are other abnormal sounds. Also note if lung and airway sounds are equal or unequal as discussed above.

Stridor

Stridor is a coarse, high-pitched sound. It is typically heard during inspiration. Sometimes stridor may be heard during both inspiration and expiration. Stridor is a sign of upper airway obstruction. It may indicate severe airway obstruction, requiring immediate intervention.

There are many causes of stridor. These include croup, aspiration of a foreign body, or infection.

Snoring

Although *snoring* may be common during sleep in children, it also can be a sign of airway obstruction. Soft tissue swelling or decreased level of consciousness may cause airway obstruction and snoring.

Barking Cough

A *barking cough* is another sign of upper airway obstruction that may occur with respiratory problems such as croup. The sound results from rapid movement of air through a narrowed upper airway.

Hoarseness

Hoarseness is a sign of upper airway obstruction caused by infection or airway swelling. Hoarseness results from swelling of the vocal cords that interferes with normal vocal sounds.

Grunting

Grunting is a short, low-pitched sound heard during expiration. Grunting may be intermittent. Sometimes it may sound like a small cry. Grunting can result from pulmonary conditions, such as pneumonia or cardiac conditions such as congestive heart failure. Grunting is typically a sign of severe respiratory distress from lung tissue disease. If grunting is present, get help.

Detailed and Advanced Concepts	Grunting occurs as the child exhales against partially closed vocal cords. Grunting increases airway pressure in an attempt to open the small airways and air sacs in the lungs. This is an effort to improve oxygenation and ventilation.

Gurgling

Gurgling is a bubbling sound heard during inspiration or expiration. It occurs when the upper airway is partially obstructed by secretions, vomit, or blood.

Wheezing

Wheezing is a high-pitched or low-pitched whistling or sighing sound heard most often during expiration. It occurs less frequently during inspiration. This sound indicates lower airway obstruction. Bronchiolitis and asthma are common causes of wheezing. Inspiratory wheezing suggests a foreign body or other obstruction in the trachea or upper airway.

Detailed and Advanced Concepts	Lower airway obstruction may be present even if you do not hear wheezing. This can happen if the child is not moving enough air with each breath. If a child is coughing and has increased respiratory rate and effort, lower airway obstruction may be present even if you do not detect a wheezing sound. In this case, the child is in severe respiratory distress and needs immediate intervention.

Crackles

Crackles are also known as rales. These are sharp, crackling sounds heard on inspiration. The sound of crackles can be described as the sound made when you rub your hair together close to your ear.

Oxygen Saturation by Pulse Oximetry

A *pulse oximeter* is a tool used to monitor the percentage of the child's hemoglobin that is saturated with oxygen. This noninvasive device can detect low oxygen saturation in a child before it causes cyanosis or bradycardia.

Detailed and Advanced Concepts	A child with cyanosis of the lips, inside the mouth, and of the nail beds has some hypoxemia (ie, an abnormally low oxygen saturation). However, not every child with a low oxygen saturation will be cyanotic. If the child is anemic, the child's hemoglobin may be too low for the cyanosis to be visible. The pulse oximeter will, however, indicate a low oxygen saturation. See "Skin Color and Temperature" in Part 7 for more information.

The pulse oximeter consists of a probe attached to the child's finger, toe, or earlobe. The probe is attached to a monitor that displays the percentage of the child's hemoglobin that is saturated with oxygen. Many pulse oximeters also show the pulse rate. Some devices have an audible warning tone that indicates decreasing oxygen saturation. Some models display the pulse signal as a waveform, so you are able to evaluate the quality of the pulse signal. For more information see "Pulse Oximetry" at the end of Part 5: "Management of Respiratory Problems."

Monitor oxygen saturation to guide your intervention.

Oxygen Saturation Reading	Intervention
94% or higher when breathing room air	Oxygenation is adequate; validate by clinical assessment
Less than 94% (hypoxemia) when breathing room air	Give supplementary oxygen
Less than 90% with supplementary oxygen (severe hypoxemia)	Get help; additional interventions are usually required, including bag-mask ventilation when level of consciousness is decreased

Interpreting Pulse Oximetry Readings

It is important to recognize that pulse oximetry indicates only the oxygen saturation of hemoglobin. It does not evaluate

- Oxygen content of the blood (ie, how much oxygen is carried by the blood)
- Oxygen delivery to the tissues
- Effectiveness of ventilation (carbon dioxide level in the blood)

The pulse oximeter requires adequate blood flow to accurately detect oxygen saturation. As a result, the pulse oximeter won't be accurate during episodes of shock or cardiac arrest. In these cases you will often get a "low signal" message. Whenever the child is in shock or cardiac arrest, your focus should be on support of the child rather than on the device.

If the pulse rate on the pulse oximeter is not the same as the heart rate on the electrocardiographic (ECG) monitor, the oxygen saturation reading may not be reliable. Immediately evaluate the child's circulation. Also, look for other signs of distress by evaluating respiratory rate, respiratory effort, and level of consciousness.

Pulse oximetry readings may be falsely high or normal in children with carbon monoxide poisoning.

Identification of Respiratory Problems

After evaluating airway and breathing, you need to identify the type and severity of any respiratory problems. This will help you provide the best interventions.

> *The earlier you detect severe respiratory distress and start appropriate intervention, the better the child's chance for a good outcome.*

Decreased Oxygenation and Ventilation in Respiratory Problems

To recognize mild and severe respiratory distress, it is helpful to understand a few basic facts about respiratory problems. This section discusses decreased oxygenation and ventilation in respiratory problems.

Function of the Respiratory System

Oxygen is taken into the lungs during inspiration. It moves from the lung air sacs (alveoli) into the blood, attaches to hemoglobin within the red blood cells, and is delivered to the body. This process is referred to as *oxygenation.* Carbon dioxide moves from the blood into the air sacs. Carbon dioxide leaves the body during expiration. The process of carbon dioxide exchange from the body through the lungs is called *ventilation.* Acute respiratory problems can result from any airway, lung tissue, or neuromuscular disease. These problems can result in low blood oxygen saturation (hypoxemia), high blood levels of carbon dioxide (poor ventilation), or both.

Infants and children have high metabolic rates. This means that they use a large amount of oxygen for each pound or kilogram of body weight as compared with adults.

Respiratory problems may result in the following conditions:

Condition	Description
Hypoxemia	Low oxygen saturation of the arterial blood
Hypercarbia	Inadequate ventilation leading to increased carbon dioxide level in the blood
Hypoxemia and hypercarbia	Low oxygen saturation and high carbon dioxide level

Low Oxygen Saturation (Hypoxemia)

Low blood oxygen saturation is called *hypoxemia.* When hypoxemia is present, the hemoglobin saturation with oxygen (often called the *oxygen saturation*) is low. Normally hemoglobin in the arterial blood is almost fully saturated (95% to 100%) with oxygen. You can detect low oxygen saturation with a pulse oximeter.

> *An oxygen saturation of less than 94% in a child breathing room air indicates hypoxemia.*

In many children hypoxemia will cause a low tissue level of oxygen (hypoxia). This can cause the child's condition to quickly worsen. Hypoxemia is only one cause of tissue hypoxia. Observe a critically ill or injured child carefully for signs of hypoxemia.

Early Signs	Late Signs
Fast respiratory rate	Slow respiratory rate, inadequate respiratory effort, apnea
Increased respiratory effort: nasal flaring, retractions	Increased respiratory effort: head bobbing, seesaw respirations, grunting
Tachycardia	Bradycardia
Pallor	Mottling, cyanosis
Agitation, anxiety	Decreased level of consciousness

Detailed and Advanced Concepts	Some children with low oxygen saturation (eg, children with cyanotic heart disease) can deliver enough oxygen to the tissues even though they are hypoxemic. These children usually have a higher than normal hemoglobin level to increase oxygen-carrying capacity within the blood. To maintain sufficient oxygen delivery, these children must have adequate heart function, blood flow, and hemoglobin level.

Inadequate Ventilation (Hypercarbia)

If the child's ventilation is inadequate, the child will develop a high level of carbon dioxide in the blood. This condition is called *hypercarbia.* Causes of hypercarbia are

- Decreased or inadequate respiratory effort
- Airway obstruction (upper or lower)
- Lung tissue disease

Detecting hypercarbia is not as simple as detecting hypoxemia. Hypoxemia is easy to evaluate by using a pulse oximeter to measure oxygen saturation of the blood; however, a pulse oximeter does not measure the amount of carbon dioxide in the blood. Also, many of the clinical signs of hypercarbia are the same as the signs of hypoxemia. One way to confirm that a child has a high level of carbon dioxide in the blood is to obtain a blood sample for blood gas analysis. You can also see if a child has high levels of carbon dioxide by end-tidal carbon dioxide monitoring.

When to Suspect Inadequate Ventilation (Hypercarbia)

Decreased level of consciousness may be an important clue that the child's ventilation may not be adequate. If hypoxemia is corrected when you give oxygen but the child's level of consciousness worsens, then the child's carbon dioxide level may be increased. With worsening hypercarbia, the child's level of consciousness may progress from irritability, agitation, or anxiety to decreased responsiveness. Get help immediately.

Identify Respiratory Problems by Type

Information from your evaluation will help you identify respiratory problems as 1 of 4 types:

- Upper airway obstruction
- Lower airway obstruction

- Lung tissue disease
- Disordered control of breathing

Respiratory problems do not always occur one at a time. A child may have more than one type of respiratory problem. For example, a child may have disordered control of breathing due to a head injury and then develop pneumonia (lung tissue disease).

Upper Airway Obstruction

Obstruction of the upper airways may occur in the nose, pharynx, larynx, and upper trachea. Obstruction can range from mild to severe. Several factors can contribute to airway obstruction in infants and children:

- A child's tongue is large in proportion to the mouth and throat. The tongue is a common cause of upper airway obstruction, particularly when a child with decreased level of consciousness lies faceup.
- An infant's head is large in proportion to the body. If an infant lies faceup on a flat surface, the neck is more likely to flex. This adds to the upper airway obstruction caused by the tongue.
- The upper airway is smaller in infants and young children. It is more easily obstructed. Infection, inflammation, or injury can cause secretions or blood to collect in the airways, nose, pharynx, and larynx. Airway obstruction can result.

Causes of Upper Airway Obstruction

Common causes of upper airway obstruction are croup, anaphylaxis, aspiration of a foreign body, or infection. Upper airway obstruction also may be caused by a medical treatment or procedure. For example, narrowing of the airway below the vocal cords may develop as a result of injury to these tissues during endotracheal intubation.

Signs of Upper Airway Obstruction

Signs of upper airway obstruction include increased respiratory rate (usually mildly elevated) and effort (eg, retractions, nasal flaring). Signs may be most apparent during inspiration. The following are signs of upper airway obstruction:

Signs of Upper Airway Obstruction
• Increased respiratory rate and effort (eg, retractions, nasal flaring)
• Decreased air movement
• Stridor (typically inspiratory)
• Barking cough
• Snoring or gurgling
• Hoarseness

Respiratory effort, chest expansion, and air movement may change rapidly, especially in infants and young children. Lung and airway sounds will change with the change in air movement. An infant or child with mild airway obstruction may rapidly progress to severe airway obstruction. When airway obstruction is severe, air movement decreases. This causes retractions and respiratory effort to increase and inspiratory sounds to disappear. You will then hear little or no air movement with a stethoscope. The child may have other signs of severe upper airway obstruction, such as drooling, increased agitation, seesaw breathing, hypoxemia, or cyanosis.

Lower Airway Obstruction

Obstruction of the lower airways may occur in the lower trachea, the bronchi, or the bronchioles.

Causes of Lower Airway Obstruction

Common causes of lower airway obstruction are

- Asthma
- Bronchiolitis

Signs of Lower Airway Obstruction

Signs of lower airway obstruction include general signs of increased respiratory rate and effort. Signs may be most apparent during expiration. The following are signs of lower airway obstruction:

Signs of Lower Airway Obstruction
- Increased respiratory rate and effort (eg, retractions, nasal flaring) - Decreased air movement - Prolonged expiration (expiration becomes an active [abnormal] process rather than a passive [normal] process) - Wheezing (heard most commonly on expiration; may also occur on both inspiration and expiration. Inspiratory wheezes alone are uncommon.)

If the child's lower airway obstruction becomes severe, the child may develop severe retractions. Decreased air movement can cause wheezing to disappear—this is an ominous finding in children with severe asthma. The child may become more agitated. If hypoxemia develops, the child may become cyanotic and lethargic.

Lung Tissue Disease

Lung tissue disease refers to a group of problems that affect lung function. In lung tissue disease the air sacs and small airways of the lungs are collapsed or filled with fluid. They no longer contain an air-oxygen mixture. Because oxygen can't move efficiently from the air sacs into the blood, children with lung tissue disease have reduced oxygen saturation in the blood. In severe lung tissue disease, ventilation is also reduced. This causes the level of carbon dioxide in the blood to rise.

Causes of Lung Tissue Disease

Some causes of lung tissue disease are

- Pneumonia: bacterial, viral, fungal, chemical
- Fluid in the lungs associated with congestive heart failure or leaking of fluids into the tissues (eg, sepsis, acute respiratory distress syndrome)
- Trauma (eg, lung bruise)
- Allergic reactions
- Toxins

Signs of Lung Tissue Disease

The following are signs of lung tissue disease:

Signs of Lung Tissue Disease
• Increased respiratory rate (often marked)
• Increased respiratory effort (especially during inspiration)
• Decreased air movement
• Grunting
• Crackles

Low oxygen saturation is usually present in lung tissue disease and may not respond to oxygen administration alone. Other advanced support (eg, endotracheal intubation, mechanical ventilation) may be needed.

Disordered Control of Breathing

Disordered control of breathing is an abnormal breathing pattern. This pattern is an *irregular* one: the child will have a normal or fast respiratory rate alternating with a slow rate or periods of apnea. Symptoms of inadequate respiratory rate, effort, or both are present. Often the parent will say the child is "breathing funny." This condition is often caused by a neurologic disorder.

Causes of Disordered Control of Breathing

Common causes of disordered control of breathing are

- Increased intracranial pressure (cerebral edema) from trauma, brain tumor, infection, or hydrocephalus
- Seizures
- Poisoning or drug overdose
- Neuromuscular disease

Increased Intracranial Pressure

Increased intracranial pressure (ICP) can be associated with a variety of conditions involving the brain. These include inflammation, infection, bleeding, trauma, tumor, and accumulation of fluid surrounding the brain.

An irregular respiratory pattern may be a sign of increased ICP. The combination of irregular breathing or apnea, a rise in blood pressure, and bradycardia suggests a life-threatening increase in ICP. Children with increased ICP, however, often have tachycardia rather than bradycardia, with irregular breathing and increased blood pressure.

Poisoning or Drug Overdose

One of the most common causes of severe respiratory distress following a poisoning or drug overdose is depression of control of breathing. A less common cause is weakness or paralysis of respiratory muscles.

Frequent complications of disordered breathing in this setting are

- Upper airway obstruction
- Decreased respiratory rate and effort
- Low oxygen saturation
- Aspiration of stomach contents or oral secretions into the lungs
- Inadequate ventilation (high level of carbon dioxide)

Neuromuscular Disease

Chronic neuromuscular disease affects the muscles of respiration. Children with these diseases commonly take very shallow breaths and do not have a strong cough. As a result, more common signs of respiratory disease, such as retractions or an increased respiratory effort, may be absent despite significant disease. These children may develop complications, including reduced clearance of secretions, collapse of the small airways and airway sacs (lung tissue), stiff lungs, and pneumonia.

Signs of Disordered Control of Breathing

The following are signs of disordered control of breathing:

Sign	Characteristic
Irregular respiratory pattern	Fast or normal rate alternating with slow rate or periods of apnea
Inadequate or irregular respiratory depth and effort	Alternating increased and inadequate respiratory effort
Normal or decreased air movement	Normal or decreased
Possible signs of upper airway obstruction	Produced by the tongue falling back into the airway, causing upper airway obstruction

Shallow breathing often causes inadequate oxygenation, ventilation, or both. Disordered control of breathing is usually caused by a condition that impairs brain function. For this reason, children with disordered control of breathing often have a decreased level of consciousness.

Identify Respiratory Problems by Severity

Respiratory distress is a clinical state characterized by abnormal respiratory rate or effort. The rate may be irregular, fast, slow, or absent. The respiratory effort may be increased (eg, nasal flaring, retractions) or inadequate (eg, apnea, weak cry or cough).

A child in respiratory distress may also have changes in chest expansion and air movement, lung and airway sounds, oxygen saturation, skin color, and level of consciousness.

Respiratory distress ranges from mild to severe. Severe respiratory distress may indicate respiratory failure. In this course students are not expected to differentiate between respiratory distress and failure. A child with severe respiratory distress needs immediate intervention.

Signs of Mild Respiratory Distress

Signs of mild respiratory distress may vary in severity. Signs may include

- Increased respiratory rate
- Increased respiratory effort (eg, nasal flaring, retractions)
- Abnormal airway and lung sounds (eg, stridor, grunting, wheezing)
- Tachycardia
- Pale, cool skin
- Changes in level of consciousness

Severe Respiratory Distress

Severe respiratory distress is defined as inadequate respiratory effort, severe increase in respiratory effort, or low oxygen saturation despite high-flow oxygen administration. If a child with severe respiratory problems does not improve or worsens, severe respiratory distress is likely present. As the child tires or as respiratory function or effort decreases, signs of severe respiratory distress develop. Be alert for the following signs of severe respiratory distress:

Signs of Severe Respiratory Distress
One or more of the following: • Very rapid or inadequate respiratory rate • Significant or inadequate respiratory effort • Low oxygen saturation despite high-flow oxygen • Bradycardia (ominous) • Cyanosis • Decreased level of consciousness

Some children with severe respiratory distress may not have signs of increased respiratory effort. This may occur in children with disordered control of breathing. *When respiratory effort is inadequate, severe respiratory distress may be present without typical signs.*

A child's condition may be identified as severe respiratory distress based on clinical findings. Laboratory tests may be required to confirm respiratory failure.

Be aware that if any child with severe respiratory distress does not improve quickly, cardiac arrest may soon follow. You must intervene quickly to prevent respiratory arrest and ultimately cardiac arrest.

Part 5

Management of Respiratory Problems

Overview

In children, respiratory problems often present before cardiac arrest. It may be very hard to decide if a child is in mild or severe respiratory distress. In children, respiratory distress can get worse very rapidly. Thus, there is little time to waste when deciding what interventions to take.

> *If severe respiratory distress is treated promptly, the child has a better chance of survival. If a child in respiratory arrest progresses to cardiac arrest, the outcome is generally poor. For the best outcome, you must intervene quickly when you identify a respiratory problem.*

This Part discusses interventions for children in mild or severe respiratory distress.

Learning Objectives

After completing this Part you should be able to

- Describe interventions to stabilize a child with mild or severe respiratory distress
- Discuss specific interventions for upper airway obstruction, lower airway obstruction, lung tissue disease, and disordered control of breathing
- Explain the use of pulse oximetry and describe its limitations

Preparation for the Course

Management of respiratory problems is a fundamental skill in caring for ill or injured children. Because management of severe respiratory problems may prevent cardiac arrest, it has significant potential to improve outcome for pediatric patients. During the course you will be expected to actively participate in case discussions, including appropriate interventions for respiratory problems. Locate the Management of Respiratory Emergencies Flowchart in the Appendix or on your PEARS Pocket Reference Card and refer to it as you study this chapter.

Management of Respiratory Distress

The primary goal for initial management of a child in mild or severe respiratory distress is to support or restore adequate oxygenation and ventilation. You build on your *evaluation* of airway and breathing to *identify* the type and severity of the respiratory problem. *Intervene* to support oxygenation and ventilation. Then repeat the evaluate-identify-intervene sequence to prioritize the next steps.

If a child is in respiratory arrest (not breathing), you must quickly identify the problem and begin rescue breathing.

Rescue Breathing

Respiratory Arrest

A child in respiratory arrest is not breathing (apnea) or is not breathing effectively but has a palpable central pulse. The provider must provide rescue breathing to prevent cardiac arrest.

Rescue Breathing

Guidelines for rescue breathing are as follows:

Rescue Breathing for Infants and Children
• Give 12 to 20 breaths/min (about 1 breath every 3 to 5 seconds).
• Give each breath in 1 second.
• Each breath should result in visible chest rise.
• Check the pulse about every 2 minutes.
• Use oxygen as soon as it is available.

If at any time you identify a life-threatening problem, immediately begin appropriate interventions. Activate emergency response as indicated in your practice setting.

Initial Management of Respiratory Distress

For a child in mild or severe respiratory distress, initial management includes some or all of the interventions listed in Table 1. Your interventions will be based on your scope of practice and local protocols. You will provide initial interventions while you gather more information to identify the type of respiratory problem that is present.

You should get help or seek expert consultation when caring for an infant or child with severe respiratory distress.

Table 1. Initial Management of Respiratory Distress

Assess	Intervention (as Indicated)

Airway	• Support the airway (allow the child to assume a position of comfort) or position the child to open the airway (perform manual airway maneuvers).
	  – If you suspect that the child may have a cervical spine injury, open the airway by using a jaw thrust without head extension.
	  – If this maneuver does not open the airway, use a head tilt with either a chin lift or a jaw thrust. Remember that opening the airway is a priority if airway obstruction is present.
	• Clear the airway (suction nose and mouth as indicated; remove a foreign body if you see it).
	• Insert an OPA as indicated.

(continued)

(continued)

Assess	Intervention (as Indicated)
Breathing	• Assess and monitor oxygenation by pulse oximetry. • Assess and monitor ventilation by evaluating respiratory rate, effort, and lung sounds. • Assist ventilation (eg, bag-mask ventilation) if needed. • Give oxygen. Provide humidified oxygen if available. Use a high-flow oxygen delivery system for severe respiratory distress. • Give medication as needed (eg, albuterol, nebulized epinephrine).
Circulation	• Monitor heart rate (note that the pulse oximeter may provide a continuous display of pulse rate; verify the reliability of this display). • Monitor level of consciousness. • Establish vascular access as needed (for fluid therapy and medications). • If the child has poor circulation, consider giving 20 mL/kg IV isotonic crystalloid (NS or LR). See Parts 7 and 8.

Abbreviations: IV, intravenous; LR, lactated Ringer's; NS, normal saline; OPA, oropharyngeal airway.

> *Remember the evaluate-identify-intervene sequence: perform frequent reevaluations.*

Interventions Based on Type of Problem

Identifying the type and severity of the child's respiratory distress will guide appropriate interventions. This Part discusses interventions for the 4 major types of respiratory problems:

- Upper airway obstruction
- Lower airway obstruction
- Lung tissue disease
- Disordered control of breathing

Management of Upper Airway Obstruction

Upper airway obstruction is a block in the large airways. Large airways include the nose, pharynx, and upper trachea. The obstruction may range from mild to severe. See "Upper Airway Obstruction" in Part 4 for more information.

General Management of Upper Airway Obstruction

General management of upper airway obstruction includes the initial interventions listed in Table 1. Additional measures focus on relieving the obstruction. These measures may include the following:

- Position the child.
  - Allow the child to assume a position of comfort.
  - If the child has a decreased level of consciousness, turn the child on his side to open the airway.
- Remove any object that you see obstructing the airway.
- Suction the nose, mouth, or both.
- Reduce airway swelling by using drugs, such as nebulized epinephrine.
- Avoid unnecessary agitation of the child, which often worsens upper airway obstruction.

Suction the airway if blood or secretions are present. *Use caution, however, if the cause of upper airway swelling is an infection (eg, croup). When swelling is present, suctioning may trigger severe coughing and laryngospasm. This may make the obstruction worse.* It may also increase the child's agitation, causing more severe respiratory distress. Allow the infant or child to assume a position of comfort. Give nebulized epinephrine if there is swelling of the upper airway.

If you recognize signs of severe upper airway obstruction, *get advanced help immediately*. A provider with skill and experience in airway management may be needed to establish an airway. Failure to aggressively treat a severe upper airway obstruction may lead to respiratory and cardiac arrest.

When severe upper airway obstruction is not present, infants and children may benefit from the use of airway adjuncts, such as an OPA. An OPA should be inserted only in an unconscious patient with no gag reflex. In the conscious child an OPA stimulates gagging and may cause vomiting.

Specific Interventions Based on Cause of Upper Airway Obstruction

Some causes of upper airway obstruction require specific interventions. This section provides information about interventions for upper airway obstruction due to the following causes:

- Croup
- Anaphylaxis
- Foreign-body airway obstruction (FBAO)

Interventions for Croup

Decide which interventions to take for croup based on your assessment of severity. Signs of croup may progress from mild to severe.

Signs of Croup	
Mild	**Severe**
Occasional barking cough	Frequent barking cough
Mild or no stridor at rest	Audible inspiratory/occasional expiratory stridor
Few or no chest retractions	Marked chest retractions
Little to no agitation	Significant agitation
Good distal air entry on auscultation	Decreased air entry on auscultation
Normal oxygen saturation	Decreased oxygen saturation (hypoxemia)

Interventions for Croup		
Mild		**Severe**
Continuously evaluate the child for signs of increasing respiratory distress	→	Get help Give nothing by mouth
Measure oxygen saturation	→	Provide high-flow oxygen Be prepared to assist ventilation with bag–mask device
Consider nebulized epinephrine	→	Administer nebulized epinephrine*
Consider steroid, such as dexamethasone	→	Administer steroid, such as dexamethasone

*Observe for at least 2 hours after giving epinephrine for "rebound" (recurrence of stridor) or increasing respiratory distress.

Interventions for Anaphylaxis

Anaphylaxis is a severe allergic reaction that requires urgent treatment. You must be able to identify if an allergic reaction is mild or severe (anaphylaxis).

Mild Allergic Reaction

Signs of a mild allergic reaction are

- Stuffy nose, sneezing, and itching around the eyes
- Itching of the skin or mucous membranes
- Raised, red rash on the skin (hives)

Interventions for Mild Allergic Reaction
Get help.
Ask the child or caregiver about any history of allergy or anaphylaxis. Look for a medical alert bracelet or necklace.
Consider an oral dose of antihistamine.

Severe Allergic Reaction (Anaphylaxis)

The signs of a severe allergic reaction are

- Trouble breathing
- Swelling of the lips, tongue, and face
- Signs of shock

In addition to the general interventions for respiratory distress listed in Table 1, *specific interventions for a severe allergic reaction (anaphylaxis)* may include the following:

Specific Interventions for Severe Allergic Reaction
Get help.
Give intramuscular epinephrine by autoinjector.* (Give a pediatric dose if the child's weight is less than 30 kg. Give an adult dose if weight is 30 kg or greater.)
The first and most important intervention in a child with moderate to severe airway obstruction due to anaphylaxis is to give IM epinephrine.

(continued)

(continued)

Specific Interventions for Severe Allergic Reaction
If wheezing is present, give albuterol by metered-dose inhaler (MDI) or nebulizer solution.
For severe respiratory distress, anticipate further airway swelling and prepare for endotracheal intubation by an advanced provider.
If hypotension is present, administer isotonic crystalloid (eg, NS or LR) 20 mL/kg IV bolus. Repeat as needed.

*Some states and local protocols permit rescuers to help children use epinephrine autoinjectors. Children who carry these devices usually know when and how to use them. You may help give the injection if you are approved to do so by state regulations and local protocols.

Interventions for Foreign-Body Airway Obstruction

In addition to the general interventions for respiratory distress listed in Table 1, *specific interventions for an FBAO* may include the following:

Interventions for a Responsive Infant or Child With FBAO	
Infant **(Less than 1 year of age)**	**Child** **(1 year to adolescent [puberty])**
1. Confirm severe airway obstruction. Check for sudden onset of severe breathing difficulty, ineffective or silent cough, weak or silent cry. 2. Give up to 5 back slaps *and* up to 5 chest thrusts. 3. Repeat Step 2 until effective or victim becomes unresponsive.	1. Ask, "Are you choking?" 2. Give abdominal thrusts/Heimlich maneuver. 3. Repeat abdominal thrusts until effective or victim becomes unresponsive.
Victim Becomes Unresponsive	
1. Send someone to activate emergency response. 2. Lower child to floor. If child is unresponsive with no breathing or only gasping, begin CPR (no pulse check). 3. Before you deliver breaths, look into the mouth. If you see a foreign body that can be easily removed, remove it. 4. Continue CPR for 5 cycles or about 2 minutes.* If you are alone, activate emergency response. Return and continue CPR until more skilled providers arrive.	

*Providing effective ventilation by using a bag-mask device during CPR to a child with an FBAO may be difficult. Consider using the 2-person bag-mask ventilation technique.

Management of Lower Airway Obstruction

Lower airway obstruction is a narrowing or blockage of the smaller airways. Smaller airways include the bronchi and bronchioles. This obstruction may be mild or severe. See "Lower Airway Obstruction" in Part 4 for more information.

General Management of Lower Airway Obstruction

In addition to the general interventions for respiratory distress listed in Table 1, *general management of lower airway obstruction* may include the following:

- Support adequate oxygenation
- Provide nebulized epinephrine or albuterol as needed
- Be prepared to support ventilation with bag-mask ventilation if needed (for severe distress)

In infants and children with severe respiratory distress, the priority is restoring adequate oxygenation and ventilation.

If bag-mask ventilation is needed for a child with lower airway obstruction, provide effective ventilation at the lower range of normal. Providing ventilation at a slow rate allows more time for expiration. This reduces the risk that air will remain inside the chest at the end of expiration. Providing too many breaths or breaths with too much volume may result in the following complications:

Complication	Result
Air enters the stomach (gastric distention)	• Increased risk of vomiting and aspiration • Can prevent adequate movement of the diaphragm, limiting effective ventilation
Risk of air leak into space surrounding the lungs	• Decreased blood flow • Risk of lung collapse from air leak into the pleural space (pneumothorax)
Severe air trapping	• Severe decrease in oxygenation • Decreased blood flow

Specific Interventions Based on Cause of Lower Airway Obstruction

Some causes of lower airway obstruction require specific interventions. This section describes interventions for lower airway obstruction due to the following causes:

- Bronchiolitis
- Acute asthma

Note: It may be difficult to decide if a wheezing infant has bronchiolitis or asthma. A history of previous wheezing episodes suggests asthma. Consider giving bronchodilators even if the diagnosis is unclear.

Interventions for Bronchiolitis

In addition to the general interventions for respiratory distress listed in Table 1, *specific interventions for bronchiolitis* may include the following:

- Perform oral or nasal suctioning as needed.
- Assist ventilation with a bag-mask device as indicated.
- Give nebulized epinephrine or albuterol by local protocol or as directed by an advanced provider.

Studies have shown that some infants with bronchiolitis improve when given nebulized epinephrine or albuterol; others do not improve or may even get worse with nebulizer therapy.

Interventions for Acute Asthma

Interventions for asthma are based on severity. Watch for the following signs that a child with asthma is getting worse:

- Decreased wheezing with continued or increasing respiratory effort
- Decreased oxygen saturation
- Decreased level of consciousness

The following table shows the progression of mild to severe signs of asthma:

Signs of Asthma		
Mild		**Severe**
May be agitated	→	Usually agitated
		Agitation progressing to decreased level of consciousness
May lie down or prefer to sit	→	Sits or leans forward
Breathless when walking	→	Breathless at rest
Talks in sentences/normal cry	→	Talks in words (infant will stop feeding)
Respiratory rate increased	→	Respiratory rate increased
Respiratory effort usually not increased	→	Respiratory effort usually increased
Moderate wheezing	→	Diminished air flow, which may result in decreased wheezing
Oxygen saturation greater than 95%	→	Oxygen saturation less than 90%
Heart rate normal to increased	→	Heart rate increased

In addition to the general interventions for respiratory distress listed in Table 1, *specific interventions for acute asthma* may include the interventions described below:

Interventions for Asthma		
Mild		**Severe**
Get help	→	Get help

(continued)

(continued)

Interventions for Asthma	
Mild	**Severe**
Give oxygen by nasal cannula or blow-by (keep oxygen saturation 94% or higher)	If oxygen saturation is 94% or higher, provide high-flow oxygen. Assist ventilation as indicated to maintain oxygen saturation 94% or higher. If oxygen saturation is less than 90% despite oxygen therapy, additional interventions (including bag-mask ventilation) are usually required. Consult with advanced providers.
Consider albuterol by MDI or nebulizer solution	Give albuterol repeatedly or by continuous nebulizer solution
Consider establishing vascular access	Establish vascular access
Administer corticosteroids PO/IV	Administer corticosteroids IV

Management of Lung Tissue Disease

Lung tissue disease is a category of respiratory problems that affect lung function. See "Lung Tissue Disease" in Part 4 for more information.

General Management of Lung Tissue Disease

General management of lung tissue disease includes the initial interventions described in Table 1. If the child is wheezing or shows other evidence of airway obstruction, interventions also may include giving a bronchodilator. Monitor clinical signs of circulation. Support as necessary.

Specific Interventions Based on Cause of Lung Tissue Disease

If the child has lung tissue disease due to infectious pneumonia, consider the following interventions:

Interventions for Infectious Pneumonia
Get help.
Give oxygen.
Draw blood cultures and administer antibiotics* (goal is to administer within first hour of medical contact).

(continued)

Interventions for Infectious Pneumonia
If wheezing is present, administer albuterol by MDI (with spacer) or nebulizer solution.
If the child has fever, take measures to reduce it.

*It may not be necessary to draw blood cultures before antibiotics are given. Follow facility protocol.

Management of Disordered Control of Breathing

Disordered control of breathing is an abnormal breathing pattern. Common causes of disordered control of breathing are neurologic problems (eg, increased ICP), poisoning or drug overdose, and neuromuscular disease. See "Disordered Control of Breathing" in Part 4 for more information.

General Management of Disordered Control of Breathing

General management of disordered control of breathing includes the initial interventions described in Table 1. Priorities are to

- Get help.
- Open the airway.
- Suction secretions if present.
- Give oxygen.
- Be prepared to provide bag-mask ventilation if respiratory rate or effort is inadequate.

Specific Interventions Based on Cause of Disordered Control of Breathing

Other interventions for specific causes of disordered control of breathing are the following:

Cause	Intervention
Increased ICP	• Get help. • Elevate the head of the bed; keep the patient's head in midline. • Treat fever. • Administer oxygen and assist ventilation with a bag-mask device.
Poisoning or drug overdose	• Get help. • If you suspect poisoning, contact your local poison control center. (In the United States, call 1-800-222-1222.) For more information on toxicology, see Parts 14 and 17 of the *2010 AHA Guidelines for CPR and ECC.* • Be prepared to suction the airway if vomiting occurs. • Be prepared to support circulation [see Part 8: "Management of Circulatory Emergencies (Shock)"].
Neuromuscular disease	• Get help. • Suction the mouth if needed; a child with neuromuscular weakness often has a weak cough and can't keep the upper airway clear.

Equipment and Procedures for Management of Respiratory Emergencies

During the PEARS Course you will need to be familiar with commonly used respiratory equipment. This section reviews the following:

Topic	Page
Bag-Mask Ventilation	51
Suctioning	59
Oropharyngeal Airway	60
Oxygen Delivery Systems	62
Respiratory Physical Exam	65
Nebulizer	66
Metered-Dose Inhaler	67
Pulse Oximetry	69

Bag-Mask Ventilation

Overview

In most emergencies when assisted ventilation is required, effective bag-mask ventilation will provide adequate oxygenation and ventilation until an advanced airway, such as an endotracheal tube, can be placed. Bag-mask ventilation can be as effective as ventilation through an endotracheal tube for short periods.

All healthcare providers who care for infants and children should be trained to deliver effective oxygenation and ventilation by using a bag-mask device as the primary method of ventilatory support.

Preparation for the Course

To successfully complete the PEARS Provider Course, you must demonstrate competency in performing bag-mask ventilation. This important skill will be evaluated in the BLS Practice and Competency Testing Station. You may also be asked to perform this skill during the cardiac arrest case simulations.

How to Select and Prepare the Equipment

A bag-mask device consists of a ventilation bag and a face mask. It can be used with or without an oxygen source. For ventilation to be effective with a bag-mask device, you must know how to select the face mask, prepare the ventilation bag, and provide supplementary oxygen if needed.

Face Mask

Select a face mask that extends from the bridge of the child's nose to the cleft of the chin, covering the nose and mouth but not compressing the eyes (Figure 1). The mask should have a soft rim (eg, flexible cuff) that molds easily to create a tight seal against the face. If the face-mask seal is not tight, oxygen intended for ventilation will escape under the mask and ventilation will not be effective.

Select a transparent mask if available. A transparent mask allows you to see the color of the child's lips and condensation on the mask (which indicates expiration). You will also be able to observe for regurgitation.

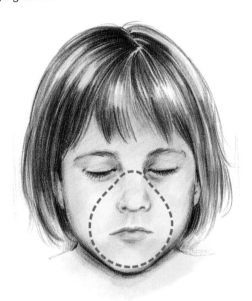

Figure 1. Proper area of the face for face-mask application. Note that no pressure is applied to the eyes.

Ventilation Bags

There are 2 types of ventilation bags: self-inflating and flow-inflating bags. Ventilation bags used for initial resuscitation are usually self-inflating. Flow-inflating bags may be used in some in-hospital settings, such as intensive care units, delivery rooms, and operating rooms. Ventilation bags come in a variety of sizes.

Oxygen Delivery

A bag-mask device may be used with or without supplementary oxygen. To deliver an inspired oxygen concentration of near 100%, attach the bag-mask device with a reservoir to an oxygen source (Figure 2, A and B). Maintain an oxygen flow of 10 to 15 L/min into the reservoir attached to a pediatric bag and a flow of at least 15 L/min into an adult bag.

> *Attach an oxygen reservoir to the self-inflating bag as soon as possible during resuscitation. Frequently verify that oxygen is attached and flowing into the bag. Remember to*
>
> - *Listen for oxygen flow*
> - *Check oxygen tank pressure or verify connection to a wall oxygen source*
> - *Verify correct flow rate*
>
> *Following resuscitation (ie, after ROSC), when an oximeter is available, titrate oxygen administration to maintain the child's oxygen saturation of 94% to 99%.*

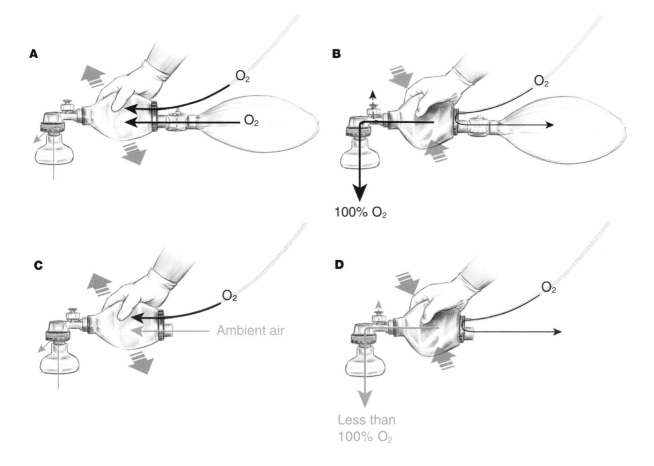

Figure 2. Self-inflating bag with (**A** and **B**) and without (**C** and **D**) an oxygen reservoir. **A,** When an oxygen reservoir is present and the bag re-expands (or refills) after it is squeezed, it fills with oxygen from the oxygen source and the oxygen reservoir. **B,** Compression of the bag provides the patient with 100% oxygen concentration. **C,** When an oxygen reservoir is not present and the bag re-expands (refills) after it is squeezed, it fills with a mixture of oxygen and ambient air. **D,** Compression of the bag provides the patient with this oxygen-air mixture.

Pop-off Valve

Check to see if the bag has a pop-off valve. Many self-inflating bags have a pressure-limited pop-off valve. This valve is set at 35 to 45 cm H_2O to prevent delivery of excessive airway pressure. Higher airway pressures may sometimes be needed for proper ventilation. If airway resistance is high, an automatic pop-off valve may prevent delivery of an effective breath that makes the chest rise. Therefore, bags used for ventilation during CPR or other emergencies should have *no pop-off valve* or the valve should be twisted into the closed position to prevent the loss of ventilation volume when high airway pressures are present. When giving ventilation with a bag-mask device, use just enough pressure to make the chest rise.

Bag Size

Use a self-inflating bag with a volume of at least 450 to 500 mL for infants and young children. Smaller bags may not deliver an adequate volume of oxygen. In older children or adolescents, you may need to use an adult self-inflating bag (1000 mL or larger) to provide effective ventilation.

How to Test the Bag-Mask Device

Check all components of the self-inflating bag and mask before use to ensure proper function. To test the device:

- Listen for an air leak: occlude the patient outlet valve with your hand and squeeze the bag.
- Check the gas flow control to verify proper function.
- Check the pop-off valve (if present) to ensure that it can be closed.
- Check that the oxygen tubing is securely connected to the device and to the oxygen source.
- Listen for the sound of oxygen flowing into the bag.
- Ensure that the cuff of the mask (if present) is adequately inflated.

How to Position the Child

Sniffing Position

Properly position the child to maintain an open airway. During bag-mask ventilation it may be necessary to move the child's head and neck gently through a range of positions to optimize ventilation. A sniffing position without hyperextension of the neck is usually best for infants and toddlers.

To achieve a sniffing position, place the child on her back. Flex the child's neck forward at the level of the shoulders while tilting the head and lifting the chin. Position the opening of the external ear canal at the level of, or in front of, the anterior aspect of the shoulder while the head is extended (Figure 3). Avoid hyperextending the neck because this may obstruct the airway.

To achieve the sniffing position, children older than 2 years may require padding under the back of the head (occiput). Younger children and infants may need padding under the shoulders or upper torso to prevent excessive flexion of the neck that can result when the prominent occiput rests on a flat surface and the neck flexes.

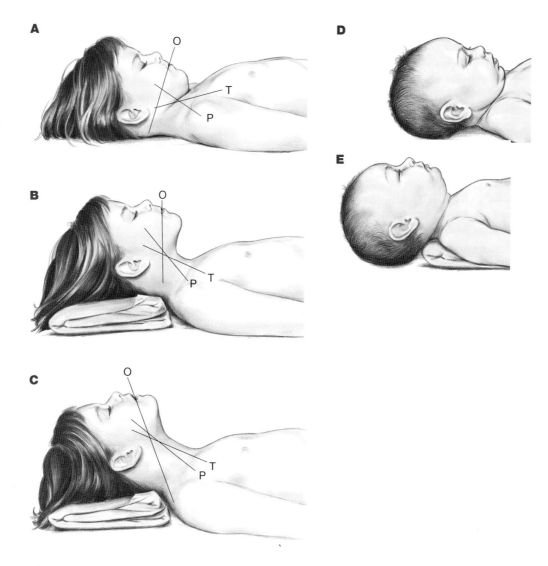

Figure 3. Positioning of a child older than 2 years for ventilation (**A-C**). **A,** With the child on a flat surface (eg, bed or table), the oral (O), pharyngeal (P), and tracheal (T) axes are misaligned. **B,** A folded sheet or towel placed under the occiput aligns the pharyngeal and tracheal axes. **C,** Extension of the neck by lifting the chin results in further alignment of the oral, pharyngeal, and tracheal axes. Note that proper positioning places the external ear canal anterior to the shoulder. Positioning of an infant (**D** and **E**). **D,** Incorrect position for an infant because of neck flexion. **E,** Correct position for an infant. Note that the external ear canal is anterior to the shoulder. Reproduced from Coté CJ, Todres ID. The pediatric airway. In: Coté CJ, Ryan JF, Todres ID, Goudsouzian NG, eds. *A Practice of Anesthesia for Infants and Children*. 2nd ed. Philadelphia, PA: WB Saunders Co; 1993:55-83, copyright Elsevier.

How to Perform Bag-Mask Ventilation

1-Person Bag-Mask Ventilation Technique

When 1 healthcare provider is performing bag-mask ventilation, the provider must open the airway and keep the mask sealed to the child's face with one hand (Figure 4) and squeeze the bag with the other hand. Effective bag-mask ventilation requires a tight seal between the mask and the child's face. Use the E-C clamp technique described below to open the airway and achieve a tight seal.

Step	Action
1	To open the airway and make a seal between the mask and the face in the absence of suspected cervical spine injury, tilt the head back. Use the E-C clamp technique to lift the jaw against the mask, pressing and sealing the mask on the face (Figure 4). This technique moves the tongue away from the posterior pharynx, moves the jaw forward, and opens the mouth. Lifting the jaw toward the mask helps seal the mask against the face. If possible, the mouth should be open under the mask, as a result of either lifting the jaw or insertion of an oropharyngeal airway. ***E-C Clamp Technique*** The technique of opening the airway and making a seal between the mask and the face is called the E-C clamp technique. The third, fourth, and fifth fingers of one hand (forming an "E") are positioned along the jaw to lift it forward; then the thumb and index finger of the same hand (forming a "C") make a seal to hold the mask to the face. Avoid pressure on the soft tissues underneath the chin (the submental area) because this can push the tongue into the posterior pharynx, resulting in airway compression and obstruction.
2	With the other hand, squeeze the ventilation bag until the chest rises. Deliver each breath over 1 second. Make sure the chest rises with each breath. Avoid excessive ventilation (see "How to Deliver Effective Ventilation" in this section).

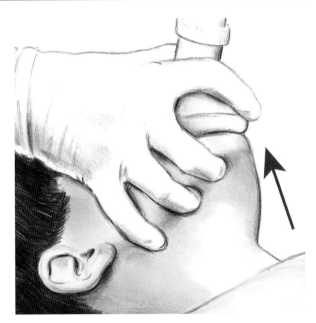

Figure 4. One-handed E-C clamp face-mask application technique. Three fingers of one hand lift the jaw (forming an "E") while the thumb and index finger hold the mask to the face (making a "C").

2-Person Bag-Mask Ventilation Technique

If 2 healthcare providers are available to perform bag-mask ventilation, one provider uses both hands to open the airway and keep the mask sealed to the child's face and the other provider squeezes the bag (Figure 5). Both providers should observe the child's chest to ensure that chest rise is visible. Be careful to avoid delivering too high a tidal volume, which may result in excessive ventilation.

The 2-person technique may provide more effective bag-mask ventilation than a 1-person technique. Also, 2-person bag-mask ventilation may be necessary when

- There is difficulty making a seal between the face and the mask
- The provider's hands are too small to reach from the front of the mask to behind the jaw or to open the airway and create a seal between the face and mask
- There is significant airway resistance (ie, asthma) or poor lung compliance (ie, pneumonia or pulmonary edema)
- Cervical spine immobilization is necessary

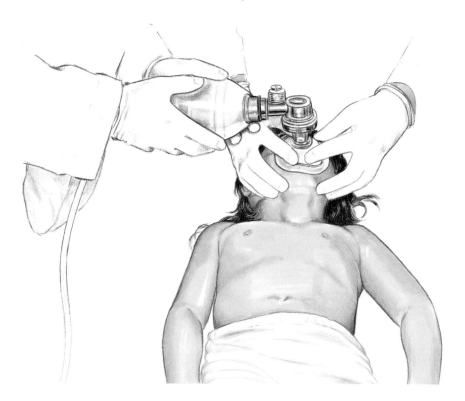

Figure 5. Two-person bag-mask ventilation technique may provide more effective ventilation than 1-person bag-mask ventilation when there is significant airway obstruction or poor lung compliance. One provider uses both hands to open the airway and maintain a tight mask-to-face seal while the other provider squeezes the ventilation bag.

How to Deliver Effective Ventilation

Precaution

Healthcare providers often deliver excessive ventilation during CPR. Excessive ventilation is harmful because it may

- Increase intrathoracic pressure, which may decrease venous return to the heart; decreased cardiac output may result
- Cause air trapping, pneumothorax, and other complications
- Increase the risk of gastric inflation and subsequent aspiration in children without an advanced airway

Clinical Parameters of Oxygenation and Ventilation

Monitor the following parameters frequently to assess the effectiveness of oxygenation and ventilation:

- Chest rise with each breath
- Oxygen saturation
- Heart rate
- Blood pressure
- Breath sounds
- Signs of improvement or deterioration (eg, appearance, color, agitation)

Troubleshooting Ineffective Ventilation

If effective ventilation is not achieved (ie, the chest does not rise), do the following:

- Reposition/reopen the airway: attempt to further lift the jaw and ensure that the child is placed in a sniffing position.
- Verify that mask size is correct.
- Ensure a tight face-mask seal.
- Suction the airway if needed.
- Check the oxygen source.
- Check the ventilation bag and mask.
- Treat gastric inflation.

Spontaneously Breathing Child

In a spontaneously breathing child, give gentle positive-pressure breaths with a bag-mask device. Time these breaths carefully to supplement the child's inspiratory efforts. If you do not coordinate the delivered breaths with the child's efforts, bag-mask ventilation may be ineffective. Poorly timed breaths may stimulate coughing, vomiting, laryngospasm, and gastric inflation, which prevent effective ventilation.

Gastric Inflation

Inflation or distention of the stomach frequently develops during bag-mask ventilation. Gastric inflation is more likely to develop during assisted ventilation if

- A partial airway obstruction is present
- High airway pressures are needed, such as in a child with poor lung compliance
- The bag-mask ventilation rate is too fast
- The volume delivered is too high
- The pressure created is too high
- The child is unconscious or is in cardiac arrest (because the gastro-esophageal sphincter opens at a lower than normal pressure)

Gastric inflation can impair a child's ventilation by limiting lung volumes.

Ways to Minimize Gastric Inflation

Minimize gastric inflation by the following:

- Ventilate at a rate of 1 breath every 3 to 5 seconds (about 12 to 20 breaths/min).
- Deliver each breath over about 1 second.
- Deliver enough volume and pressure to produce visible chest rise.

Note: There is insufficient evidence to recommend the routine use of cricoid pressure application to prevent aspiration.

Advanced providers may perform gastric decompression by inserting a nasogastric (NG) or orogastric (OG) tube.

Suctioning

Preparation for the Course

You may need to use a suction device to remove secretions (eg, blood, vomit), according to your scope of practice.

Suction Devices

Suction devices can be either portable or wall-mounted units.

- Portable suction devices are easy to transport. They may not have adequate suction power, however. A suction force of −80 to −120 mm Hg is generally needed to remove airway secretions.
- Bulb or syringe suction devices are simple to use and require no outside vacuum source. These devices may be inadequate in larger patients or when secretions are thick or copious.
- Wall-mounted suction units can provide high suction force of more than −300 mm Hg.

Suction devices used in children should have adjustable suction regulators so that you can use sufficient suction force and minimize tissue trauma. Large-bore, noncollapsible suction tubing should always be joined to the suction unit. Semirigid pharyngeal tips (tonsil suction tips) and appropriate sizes of catheters should be available.

Indications

Suctioning of secretions, blood, or vomit from the oropharynx, nasopharynx, or trachea may be needed to achieve or maintain a patent airway.

Complications

Complications of suctioning can include

- Hypoxemia
- Vagal stimulation resulting in bradycardia
- Gagging and vomiting
- Soft tissue injury
- Agitation

Soft vs Rigid Catheters

Both soft flexible and rigid suctioning catheters are available.

Use	For
A soft flexible plastic suction catheter	• Aspiration of thin secretions from the oropharynx and nasopharynx • Suctioning an advanced airway (eg, endotracheal tube)
A rigid wide-bore suction cannula ("tonsil tip")	• Suctioning of the oropharynx, particularly if thick secretions, vomit, or blood is present

Catheter Sizes

For a guide to selecting the appropriate size suction catheter, use a color-coded length-based resuscitation tape or other reference.

Oropharyngeal Suctioning Procedure

Follow the steps below to suction the oropharynx.

Step	Intervention
1	Gently insert the distal end of the suction catheter or device into the oropharynx over the tongue. Guide it into the posterior pharynx (back of the throat).
2	Apply suction by covering the catheter side opening. At the same time withdraw the catheter with a rotating or twisting motion.
3	Try to limit suction attempts to 10 seconds. This will help reduce the risk of hypoxemia (low oxygen saturation). You may give short periods of 100% oxygen immediately before and after each suctioning attempt. *Note:* Suction attempts may need to be longer than 10 seconds if the airway is obstructed (eg, by blood). You cannot provide adequate oxygenation or ventilation unless the airway is open and clear.

> *Monitor the child's heart rate, oxygen saturation, and clinical appearance during suctioning. In general, if bradycardia develops or clinical appearance deteriorates, interrupt suctioning. Give high-flow oxygen until the heart rate and clinical appearance return to normal.*

Oropharyngeal Airway

Preparation for the Course

During the course you will have an opportunity to practice using an oropharyngeal airway (OPA).

Description

The OPA consists of a flange, a short bite-block segment, and a curved body. The curved body is usually made of plastic. It is shaped to provide an air channel and a passage for a suction catheter to the pharynx. The OPA fits over the tongue to prevent it and other soft structures of the throat from obstructing the airway. An OPA is not intended to be used long term as a bite-block device in agitated patients.

Indications

An OPA may relieve upper airway obstruction caused by the tongue. If an OPA of correct size is used (see below), it will not damage laryngeal structures. An OPA may be used in the *unconscious* child with no gag reflex if procedures to open the airway (eg, head tilt–chin lift or jaw thrust) fail to provide and maintain a clear, unobstructed airway. An OPA should *not* be used in a *conscious* or *semiconscious* child because it may stimulate gagging and vomiting. Before using an OPA, check to see if the child has a gag reflex. If so, do not use an OPA.

Complications

It is important to choose the correct size OPA. If the OPA is *too large*, it can block the airway or cause trauma to the laryngeal structures (Figure 6C).

If the OPA is *too small* or is inserted improperly, it can cause the tongue to obstruct the airway (Figure 6D).

Airway Selection and Insertion Procedure

OPA sizes range from 4 to 10 cm in length (Guedel sizes 000 to 4). Follow the steps below to choose the correct size OPA and insert it into the airway.

Step	Action
1	Place the OPA against the side of the child's face (Figure 6A). The tip of the OPA should extend from the corner of the mouth to the angle of the jaw (Figure 6B).
2	Gently insert the OPA directly into the oropharynx. The use of a tongue blade to depress the tongue may be helpful.
3	After insertion of an OPA, monitor the child. Keep the head and jaw positioned properly to maintain a patent airway. Suction the airway as needed.

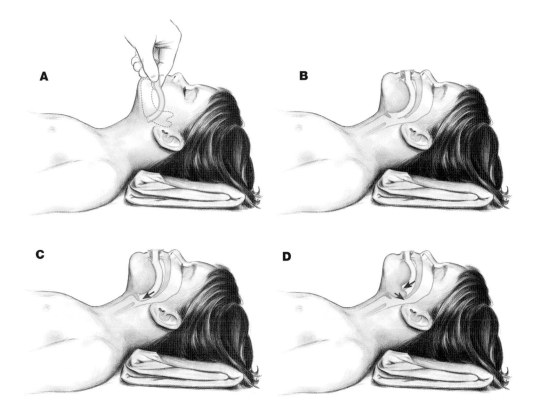

Figure 6. Selection of an OPA. A properly sized OPA relieves airway obstruction caused by the tongue without damaging the larynx. To select the proper size, hold the airway next to the child's face (**A**). The tip of the OPA should end just at the angle of the jaw, so that once inserted, it will align with the glottic opening (**B**). If it is too large (**C**), the OPA will obstruct the airway by pushing the epiglottis down (**C,** arrow). If it is too small (**D**), the OPA will worsen airway obstruction by pushing the tongue into the lower part of the throat (**D,** arrows). Adapted from Coté CJ, Todres ID. The pediatric airway. In: Coté CJ, Ryan JF, Todres ID, Goudsouzian NG, eds. *A Practice of Anesthesia for Infants and Children*. 2nd ed. Philadelphia, PA: WB Saunders Co; 1993:55-83, copyright Elsevier.

Oxygen Delivery Systems

Preparation for the Course

To be successful in the PEARS Provider Course, you will need to understand how and when to use different oxygen delivery systems. During the course you will watch a video demonstration of the correct use of oxygen delivery devices. These devices include a nasal cannula, simple oxygen mask, and nonrebreathing mask with reservoir. You will need to know the correct oxygen flow rates to use for each delivery device.

Indications for Oxygen

For children with respiratory distress or shock, oxygen uptake by the lungs and oxygen delivery to the tissues are typically reduced. At the same time tissue demand for oxygen may be increased. Give high-flow oxygen to all seriously ill or injured children with severe respiratory distress, shock, or changes in mental status. As soon as possible, add humidification to the oxygen delivery system. This may help prevent airway dryness.

Giving Oxygen to a Conscious Child

When giving oxygen to an alert child in respiratory distress, balance the need to improve oxygen delivery against the possible agitation that may result from applying an oxygen delivery device. Agitation can increase oxygen demand and respiratory distress. If a child is agitated by one method of oxygen delivery, try an alternative technique. For example, if the child is upset by an oxygen mask, try directing a "blow-by" stream of humidified oxygen toward the child's mouth and nose. It may be helpful to have a person familiar to the child, such as a parent, introduce the oxygen delivery equipment.

When giving oxygen to an alert child in respiratory distress, allow the child to remain in a position of comfort. This will minimize respiratory effort and help keep the airway as open as possible. For infants and young children, the best position might be in the arms of the parent or caregiver.

Giving Oxygen to a Child With a Decreased Level of Consciousness

If a child has a decreased level of consciousness, the airway may become obstructed by a combination of the following:

- Flexion of the neck
- Relaxation of the jaw
- Displacement of the tongue against the back of the throat

If the child is unconscious with no cough or gag reflex, open the airway and insert an oropharyngeal airway. Use the head tilt–chin lift maneuver or a jaw thrust to open the airway.

> *A properly performed jaw thrust is the most effective means to open the pediatric airway. Providers, however, are often inexperienced with this technique because it is difficult to practice the skill with some CPR manikins.*

If no trauma is suspected and the child is breathing normally, roll the child onto her side in a neutral position. Place the child on her side only if no other interventions are needed.

Suction the oropharynx and nasopharynx to clear secretions, mucus, or blood if needed. Once the airway is open and clear, you can give oxygen by a variety of oxygen delivery systems.

Types of Oxygen Delivery Systems

For a spontaneously breathing child who needs supplementary oxygen, you need to know which oxygen delivery system to use. Oxygen delivery systems are either low flow or high flow. Consider the child's clinical status and the desired concentration of inspired oxygen when choosing the appropriate system.

Oxygen Delivery System	Device
Low-flow oxygen	• Nasal cannula • Simple oxygen mask
High-flow oxygen	• Nonrebreathing mask with reservoir

The concentration of inspired oxygen is determined by several factors. These include oxygen flow into the device, the child's inspiratory flow, and how tightly the device fits against the child's face.

Low-Flow Oxygen Delivery Systems

A low-flow oxygen delivery system delivers air through a nasal cannula or a simple mask that does not fit tightly against the child's face. The oxygen flow into the delivery device is less than the child's inspiratory flow rate. When the child inhales, the child inspires some room air in addition to the oxygen provided by the device. As a result, the oxygen from the device mixes with room air, so a variable concentration of oxygen is delivered to the child. The higher the oxygen flow provided, the higher the inspired oxygen concentration.

Low-flow systems generally provide an inspired oxygen concentration of about 22% to 60%. Low-flow oxygen systems are used when the child requires a relatively low inspired oxygen concentration and is relatively stable, such as when the child is not in severe respiratory distress or shock.

The nasal cannula and simple oxygen mask are examples of low-flow oxygen delivery systems.

Nasal Cannula

The nasal cannula is typically a low-flow oxygen delivery device. It delivers an inspired oxygen concentration of 22% to 60%. The appropriate oxygen flow rate for the nasal cannula is 0.25 to 4 L/min.

The nasal cannula is suitable for infants and children who require only low levels of supplementary oxygen. Note that in small infants a nasal cannula may deliver a high inspired oxygen concentration. The inspired oxygen concentration delivered via nasal cannula cannot be reliably determined from the oxygen flow rate alone. It is also influenced by other factors, such as

- The child's size
- Inspiratory flow rate
- Volume of inspired air
- Nasopharyngeal and oropharyngeal volume
- Nasal resistance (eg, oxygen delivery is compromised if nares are obstructed)
- Oropharyngeal resistance

Delivery of a high oxygen flow rate (greater than 4 L/min) through a nasal cannula irritates the nasopharynx. This rate also may not improve oxygenation. A nasal cannula often does not provide humidified oxygen.

Simple Oxygen Mask

The simple oxygen mask is a low-flow device. It delivers an inspired oxygen concentration of 35% to 60%. The appropriate flow rate for the simple oxygen mask is 6 to 10 L/min.

The simple oxygen mask cannot deliver an inspired oxygen concentration greater than 60%. This is because room air enters the mask between the mask and the face and through ports in the side of the mask during inspiration. The oxygen concentration delivered to the child is reduced if

- The child's inspiratory flow is high
- The mask does not fit tightly against the face
- The oxygen flow into the mask is low

A minimum oxygen flow rate of 6 L/min is needed to maintain an increased inspired oxygen concentration and prevent rebreathing of exhaled carbon dioxide.

There are several types of oxygen masks that can deliver humidified oxygen in a wide range of concentrations. The soft vinyl pediatric mask may cause infants and toddlers to become agitated and upset. This increases oxygen demand and could result in increased respiratory distress. This mask may be used effectively in older children.

High-Flow Oxygen Delivery Systems

High-flow oxygen systems reliably deliver a high concentration of oxygen of greater than 60%. In a high-flow oxygen delivery system the oxygen flow rate is high, at least 10 L/min. An oxygen reservoir is present and fills with oxygen to meet the total maximum inspired flow requirements of the child. Room air does not enter the mask if the mask is tight-fitting and the delivery system is closed.

High-flow systems should be used in emergency settings whenever the child has respiratory distress or shock. A nonrebreathing mask is the most common example of a high-flow system.

Nonrebreathing Mask

The nonrebreathing mask (Figure 7) is a high-flow delivery device. An inspired oxygen concentration of 95% can be achieved with an oxygen flow rate of 10 to 15 L/min and the use of a well-sealed face mask.

A nonrebreathing mask consists of a face mask and reservoir bag with the addition of 2 valves:

- A valve in one exhalation port to prevent room air from entering the mask during inspiration
- A valve placed between the reservoir bag and the mask to prevent the flow of exhaled gas into the reservoir

Adjust the oxygen flow rate into the mask to prevent collapse of the bag. During inspiration the child draws 100% oxygen from the reservoir bag and the oxygen inflow.

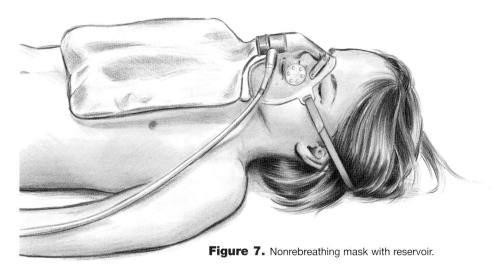

Figure 7. Nonrebreathing mask with reservoir.

Respiratory Physical Exam

Preparation for the Course

You may need to know the auscultation points for a respiratory physical exam, according to your scope of practice.

Auscultation With a Stethoscope

Use a stethoscope to auscultate the following points during a respiratory physical exam:

- Anterior (on either side of the breastbone)
- Posterior
- Lateral (under the axillae)

For more information, see "Chest Expansion and Air Movement" in Part 4.

Nebulizer

Preparation for the Course

Inhaled medications can be delivered via a nebulizer. The nebulizer is a device that uses compressed air or oxygen to deliver liquid medication as a fine mist. The child then inhales the mist into his lungs.

You may need to know how to assemble a nebulizer, set correct oxygen flow, and give nebulized medications if these tasks are within your scope of practice. You should be familiar with the operation of the nebulizer equipment used in your workplace.

Components

A nebulizer has the following components:

- Nebulizer reservoir
- Nebulizer cap
- T-piece
- Spacer
- Handheld mouthpiece or face mask
- Plastic oxygen tubing
- Oxygen source or compressed air

Older children may use the handheld mouthpiece instead of the face mask.

Steps for Using a Nebulizer With a Handheld Mouthpiece

General steps for using a nebulizer with a handheld mouthpiece (Figure 8) are as follows:

Step	Action
1	Unscrew the cap of the nebulizer reservoir. Add medication (eg, albuterol) to the nebulizer reservoir. Reattach the cap.
2	Connect the T-piece to the top of the nebulizer reservoir.
3	Connect the spacer to one end of the T-piece.
4	Connect the mouthpiece to the other end of the T-piece.
5	Connect plastic tubing between the bottom of the nebulizer bottle and the pressurized oxygen/gas source.
6	Set the gas flow at 5 to 6 L/min.
7	Hold the nebulizer reservoir upright during delivery of the medication through the mouthpiece. • Place the mouthpiece in the child's mouth and show him how to hold it. • Tell the child, "Take long, slow, deep breaths through your mouth." Continue the treatment (about 8 to 10 minutes) until the nebulizer reservoir is empty and no mist flows from the T-piece.

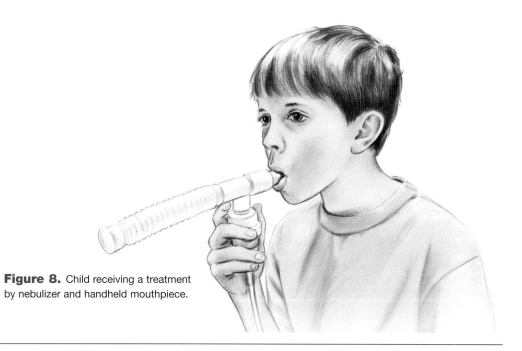

Figure 8. Child receiving a treatment by nebulizer and handheld mouthpiece.

Steps for Using a Nebulizer With a Face Mask

Step	Action
1	Unscrew the cap of the nebulizer reservoir. Add medication (eg, albuterol) to the nebulizer reservoir. Reattach the cap.
2	Attach the face mask to the top of the nebulizer reservoir.
3	Connect plastic tubing between the bottom of the nebulizer reservoir and the pressurized oxygen/gas source.
4	Set the gas flow at 5 to 6 L/min.
5	Hold the nebulizer reservoir upright during delivery of the medication through a face mask. • Place the face mask over the child's face so that it covers both the nose and mouth. Press the mask to the face to ensure a tight seal. • Tell the child, "Take long, slow, deep breaths through your mouth." Continue the treatment (about 8 to 10 minutes) until the nebulizer bottle is empty and no mist flows from the T-piece.

Metered-Dose Inhaler

Preparation for the Course

You may need to know the correct technique for helping a child use a metered-dose inhaler (MDI), according to your scope of practice. An MDI is a handheld device that delivers a dose of medicine. This dose may also be referred to as a *puff*.

This section discusses using an MDI with a spacer device (with and without a face mask). Using an MDI with a spacer device is the best method to optimize drug delivery to the lung.

Using an MDI With a Spacer Device

Follow these steps to use an MDI with a spacer device (with and without a face mask).

Step	Action
1	Remove the cap from the spacer. Insert the mouthpiece of the MDI into the rubber-sealed end of the spacer device. Attach the mouthpiece to the other end. Once assembled, shake the inhaler and spacer about 5 times.
2	Tell the child to exhale. Place the mouthpiece of the spacer device into the child's mouth (Figure 9). *or* If you are using a spacer device with a face mask, place the mask over the child's face so that it covers both the nose and the mouth (Figure 10). Press the mask to the face to ensure a tight seal. **Figure 9.** Child self-administering a treatment by MDI with a spacer device. **Figure 10.** Child receiving a treatment by MDI with a mask spacer device.

(continued)

(continued)

Step	Action
3	Press down on the inhaler to release the medication into the spacer device. Tell the child to take a very slow deep breath through the mouth-piece and hold that breath for 10 seconds. *or* If you are using a spacer device with a face mask, depress the inhaler and allow the child to breathe normally through the mask for 3 to 5 breaths per release of medication.

Pulse Oximetry

Preparation for the Course

In the PEARS Provider Course and course materials there are many references to measuring oxygen saturation by pulse oximetry. Review the section "Oxygen Saturation by Pulse Oximetry" in Part 4 for basic information about this monitoring method.

When to Use Pulse Oximetry

When caring for a seriously ill or injured child, use pulse oximetry to monitor

- Oxygen saturation
- Trends in oxygen saturation

> *Oxygen saturation is the percent of hemoglobin that is saturated with oxygen. This saturation does not equate to oxygen delivery to the tissues. It is also important to note that oxygen saturation does not provide information about effectiveness of ventilation (carbon dioxide elimination).*

Confirm the Validity of Oximeter Data

The pulse oximeter requires pulsatile blood flow to determine oxygen saturation. Different brands of pulse oximeters vary in how quickly they reflect the development of hypoxemia and in their accuracy when the child has decreased blood flow; all are inaccurate unless the pulse rate displayed by the oximeter is consistent with the heart rate displayed by the cardiac monitor. Note that skin pigment does not affect the accuracy or function of the pulse oximeter.

> *Confirm the validity of oximeter data by evaluating the child's appearance. Also compare the heart rate displayed by the pulse oximeter with the heart rate on the bedside cardiorespiratory monitor or from physical examination.*
>
> *You should immediately evaluate the child if the oximeter*
>
> - *Fails to detect a signal*
> - *Displays an inaccurate pulse rate*
> - *Indicates a weak signal*
> - *Indicates a fall in oxygen saturation*
>
> *If the oximeter fails to detect a signal or indicates a fall in oxygen saturation, you should immediately evaluate the child. Do not assume that the pulse oximeter is malfunctioning.*

The pulse oximeter may not be functioning correctly if

- The displayed heart rate does not correlate with the child's heart rate
- The child's appearance does not correspond with the reported level of oxygen saturation

Accuracy of Readings in Clinical Settings

Pulse oximetry can accurately estimate oxygen saturation but does not provide evidence of oxygen delivery. It also does not directly evaluate the effectiveness of ventilation (carbon dioxide level).

Pulse oximetry may be inaccurate in the following settings:

Setting	Cause/Solution
Cardiac arrest	Cause: Absence of blood flow Solution: None. Many devices will not be useful during cardiac arrest.
Shock or hypothermia	Cause: Decreased blood flow Solution: Improve blood flow (treat the shock). You may be able to find an alternative site (particularly one that is closer to the heart) where the device can detect a pulse.
Motion, shivering, or bright overhead lighting	Cause: False signals and inaccurate oxygen saturation values Solution: Move the sensor unit closer to the heart. Lightly cover the device in position (ie, if it is placed on a finger, lightly cover the finger to reduce ambient light).
Problem with the skin probe interface	Cause: Low or absent pulse signals Solution: Try an alternate site or alternate skin probe.
Misalignment of sensor with light source	Cause: Low or absent pulse signals Solution: Reposition the device so that the light source is located directly across the tissue bed from the sensor.
Cardiac arrhythmias with low cardiac output	Cause: Arrhythmias interfere with detection of a pulse and calculation of pulse rate Solution: Get help to treat the arrhythmia.

Correct Use of Equipment

Correct probe positioning is critical for accurate oxygen saturation readings. The probe is typically applied to a finger or toe. Falsely low readings can occur when the probe is not positioned correctly. Repositioning of the probe can result in immediate improvement in the detection of oxygen saturation by the device.

In addition to applying the probe to a finger or toe, the following locations can be used to solve placement problems.

If	Use
Infant probes are unavailable	Use an adult probe around the hand or foot of an infant.
Blood flow is significantly reduced and no signal is detected in the extremities	Apply an infant probe to the earlobe.

Pulse oximetry equipment should be used as follows:

- Use compatible equipment as recommended by the manufacturer. Do not mix the probes of one manufacturer with the computerized units of another.
- Do not use a probe with a cracked surface because the light source may come in contact with the skin and cause a burn.

Part 6

Respiratory Case Discussions

Respiratory Case Discussions (Respiratory Cases 1-4)

During the course you will watch short videos* of seriously ill or injured children with respiratory problems. Your instructor will lead the group in a discussion of the PEARS Systematic Approach for each case. These discussions will follow the format outlined below.

*To help improve your assessment skills, the PEARS Course includes videos of actual children with medical problems that you may encounter. These videos may be disturbing to some viewers. In some cases videos were looped or edited to provide you with adequate assessment time and to emphasize key teaching points.

At no time was medical care delayed for the purpose of obtaining video footage. All of these children received timely and appropriate medical care, mainly in children's hospitals. Consent was obtained before any video recording.

Initial Impression

Remember that the initial impression is your first quick (in a few seconds) "from the doorway" observation of the following:

Consciousness	Level of consciousness (eg, unresponsive, irritable, alert)
Breathing	Increased work of breathing, absent or decreased respiratory effort, or abnormal sounds heard without a stethoscope
Color	Abnormal skin color, such as pallor, mottling, or cyanosis

The purpose is to quickly identify a life-threatening problem.

Unresponsive or Responsive?

Is the child unresponsive with no breathing or only gasping? If so, provide emergency treatment and activate emergency response as appropriate in your setting.

If the child is responsive, continue the evaluate-identify-intervene sequence.

Continue the Evaluate-Identify-Intervene Sequence

Use the **evaluate-identify-intervene** sequence when caring for a seriously ill or injured child.

- *Evaluate* the child to gather information about the child's condition or status.
- *Identify* any problem by type and severity.
- *Intervene* with appropriate actions to treat the problem.

Then repeat the sequence; this process is ongoing.

Evaluate

Evaluate by using the primary assessment. In the respiratory cases you will only evaluate airway and breathing:

Airway

Clear	Maintainable	Not maintainable

Breathing

Respiratory Rate and Pattern	Respiratory Effort		Chest Expansion and Air Movement	Abnormal Lung and Airway Sounds		Oxygen Saturation by Pulse Oximetry
Normal	Normal	Inadequate	Normal	Stridor	Gurgling	Normal oxygen saturation (≥94%)
Irregular	Increased	• Apnea	Decreased	Snoring	Wheezing	
Fast	• Nasal flaring	• Weak cry or cough	Unequal	Barking cough	Crackles	Hypoxemia (<94%)
Slow	• Retractions		Prolonged expiration	Hoarseness	Unequal	
Apnea	• Head bobbing			Grunting		
	• Seesaw respirations					

Identify by Type and Severity

	Type	Severity
Respiratory	• Upper airway obstruction • Lower airway obstruction • Lung tissue disease • Disordered control of breathing	• Mild respiratory distress • Severe respiratory distress

Identifying Respiratory Problems		
Signs	**Type of Problem**	**Severity**

• Increased respiratory rate and effort (eg, retractions, nasal flaring)
• Decreased air movement
• Stridor (typically inspiratory)
• Barking cough
• Snoring or gurgling
• Hoarseness
	Upper airway obstruction	**Mild respiratory distress**
		
		• Some abnormal signs, but no signs of severe distress
		  – Increased respiratory rate
		  – Increased respiratory effort
		  – Abnormal airway and lung sounds
		  – Tachycardia
		  – Pale, cool skin
		  – Changes in level of consciousness

• Increased respiratory rate and effort (eg, retractions, nasal flaring) • Decreased air movement • Prolonged expiration • Wheezing	**Lower airway obstruction**	**Severe respiratory distress** *One or more of the following:*
• Increased respiratory rate and effort • Decreased air movement • Grunting • Crackles	**Lung tissue disease**	• Very rapid or inadequate respiratory rate • Significant or inadequate respiratory effort • Low oxygen saturation despite high-flow oxygen
• Irregular respiratory pattern • Inadequate or irregular respiratory depth and effort • Normal or decreased air movement • Possible signs of upper airway obstruction (see above)	**Disordered control of breathing**	• Bradycardia (ominous) • Cyanosis • Decreased level of consciousness

Intervene

For a quick reference on management of respiratory problems, see the Management of Respiratory Emergencies Flowchart on your PEARS Pocket Reference Card or in the Appendix.

For more details, see the following sections in Part 5: "Management of Respiratory Problems":

For	See
Initial management of respiratory problems	Table 1. Initial Management of Respiratory Distress
Upper airway obstruction	General Management of Upper Airway Obstruction Specific Interventions Based on Cause of Upper Airway Obstruction
Lower airway obstruction	General Management of Lower Airway Obstruction Specific Interventions Based on Cause of Lower Airway Obstruction

(continued)

(continued)

For	See
Lung tissue disease	General Management of Lung Tissue Disease Specific Interventions Based on Cause of Lung Tissue Disease
Disordered control of breathing	General Management of Disordered Control of Breathing Specific Interventions Based on Cause of Disordered Control of Breathing

Case 1 Notes

Case 2 Notes

Case 3 Notes

Case 4 Notes

Part 7

Circulation, Disability, and Exposure: Primary Assessment and Identification of Shock

Overview

As we discussed in Part 2: "PEARS Systematic Approach to the Seriously Ill or Injured Child," the primary assessment is a hands-on evaluation of

- **A**irway
- **B**reathing
- **C**irculation
- **D**isability
- **E**xposure

Airway and breathing were discussed in Part 4. In this Part we will focus on circulation, disability, and exposure.

> *Important: If at any time you identify a life-threatening problem, immediately begin appropriate interventions. Activate emergency response as indicated in your practice setting. Continue the primary assessment only after life-threatening problems have been addressed.*

Learning Objectives

After completing this Part you should be able to

- Summarize the CDE components of the primary assessment
- Evaluate respiratory and/or circulatory problems by using the ABCDE model
- Define shock
- Describe how to evaluate signs of circulation and recognize signs of poor perfusion
- Differentiate between compensated shock and hypotensive shock
- Recognize clinical signs and symptoms of hypovolemic and distributive shock

Preparation for the Course

A systematic approach using the primary assessment is a fundamental concept in the PEARS Course. As you study this chapter, refer to the PEARS Systematic Approach Summary located in the Appendix and on your PEARS Pocket Reference Card.

Primary Assessment: Circulation, Disability, and Exposure

Circulation

C

Evaluate Circulation

To assess circulation, evaluate

- Heart rate
- Pulses (both peripheral and central)
- Capillary refill time
- Skin color and temperature
- Blood pressure

The child's level of consciousness will help you evaluate blood flow to the brain. Urine output can also help you evaluate blood flow to the kidneys. During the PEARS Course you will use your evaluation of circulation to identify *signs of poor perfusion*.

> *Use information gathered from your evaluation of circulation to identify signs of poor perfusion: weak peripheral pulses, delayed capillary refill time, changes in skin color (pale, mottled, or cyanotic), cool skin, decreased level of consciousness, and decreased urine output.*

Heart Rate

To determine heart rate, check the pulse rate, listen to the heart, or view a monitor (ECG monitor or pulse oximeter display). Attach a 3-lead ECG monitoring system when practical.

The heart rate should be appropriate for the child's age, level of activity, and clinical condition (Table 1). Note that there is a wide range for normal heart rates. For example, a child who is sleeping or is athletic may have a heart rate lower than the normal range for age. A child with a fever, especially a high fever, should have a faster heart rate.

The heart rhythm is typically regular with only small fluctuations in rate.

> *Get help if a child's heart rate is outside the normal range or if the heart rate is not appropriate for the child's clinical condition.*

Normal Heart Rate

Table 1. Normal Heart Rates (per Minute) by Age

Age	Awake Rate	Mean	Sleeping Rate
Newborn to 3 months	85 to 205	140	80 to 160
3 months to 2 years	100 to 190	130	75 to 160
2 years to 10 years	60 to 140	80	60 to 90
Older than 10 years	60 to 100	75	50 to 90

Modified from Gillette PC, Garson A Jr, Crawford F, Ross B, Ziegler V, Buckles D. Dysrhythmias. In: Adams FH, Emmanouilides GC, Reimenschneider TA, eds. *Moss' Heart Disease in Infants, Children, and Adolescents*. 4th ed. Baltimore, MD: Williams & Wilkins; 1989:925-939.

Abnormal Heart Rate

An *abnormal heart rate* is defined as a heart rate that is either too fast (tachycardia) or too slow (bradycardia). It is best to assess the heart rate when the child is resting.

Tachycardia

Tachycardia is a heart rate that is faster than normal for age. A heart rate that is 220 per minute or higher in infants or 180 per minute or higher in children may be one sign of a life-threatening condition.

When the heart rate is too fast, the ventricles may not fill completely with blood between contractions. This may result in inadequate blood flow. Tachycardia is a common, nonspecific sign of distress. It can develop in response to many problems. Tachycardia is often appropriate when the child is seriously ill or injured. However, tachycardia may indicate a rhythm problem.

Detailed and Advanced Concepts	Tachycardia can be a normal response or can be abnormal. Sinus tachycardia and tachycardia caused by an abnormal rhythm are 2 types of tachycardia in children. Providers need information from the child's history, physical examination, and ECG analysis to determine the type of tachycardia.
	Sinus tachycardia is a rapid heart rate that originates in the natural pacemaker of the heart. It may occur as a normal response to anxiety, exertion, fear, exercise, or pain. Sinus tachycardia may also develop in a child with fever, low oxygen delivery (eg, anemia), dehydration, shock, or respiratory distress. If a child has sinus tachycardia, quickly evaluate for signs of shock and respiratory problems.
	Tachycardia can also result from an abnormal rhythm. The abnormal rate and rhythm may cause signs of shock, heart failure, or even cardiac arrest.

Bradycardia

Bradycardia is a heart rate that is slower than normal for age. When the heart beats too slowly, the heart may not pump enough blood. Bradycardia may be normal in athletic adolescents, but bradycardia with low blood pressure or poor circulation is never normal. In such cases, bradycardia could indicate that the child may soon develop cardiac arrest.

Severe respiratory distress and inadequate oxygenation of the blood are most common causes of bradycardia in a child.

If a child with bradycardia...	Then...
Has decreased responsiveness or other signs of poor perfusion	Immediately support ventilation and provide oxygen. Be prepared to start chest compressions.
Is alert, responsive, and has no signs of poor perfusion	Consider other causes of slow heart rate, such as heart block or drug overdose. Note that a slow heart rate may be normal in athletic adolescents.

Pulses

Evaluation of pulses is an important part of the assessment of circulation. Feel both the central and peripheral pulses.

Central Pulses	Peripheral Pulses
• Femoral • Carotid (in older children)	• Radial • Brachial • Dorsalis pedis • Posterior tibial

In healthy infants and children (unless the child is obese or in a cold environment), you should be able to palpate these pulses easily.

> *If you suspect that cardiac arrest is present in an unresponsive child with no breathing or only gasping, attempt to palpate a central rather than a peripheral pulse. Attempt to palpate the brachial pulse in an infant and the carotid or femoral pulse in a child.*

Central pulses are stronger than peripheral pulses. This is because these blood vessels are larger and closer to the heart. The difference in quality between central and peripheral pulses is exaggerated when small blood vessels constrict with shock.

In shock, blood flow (ie, perfusion) often decreases. The decrease in perfusion starts in the hands and feet with loss of peripheral pulses. It then extends toward the trunk, with eventual weakening of central pulses. A cold environment can also constrict the blood vessels. This constriction can cause a difference in volume between peripheral and central pulses. Central pulses, however, should remain strong.

> *Weak central pulses are a worrisome sign that the child requires very rapid intervention to prevent cardiac arrest. Call for help and support airway, oxygenation, and breathing. Be prepared to obtain immediate vascular access or give a fluid bolus.*

Capillary Refill Time

Capillary refill time is the time it takes for blood to return to tissue that has been blanched with pressure. Normal capillary refill time is 2 seconds or less. Capillary refill reflects circulation to the skin. Abnormalities in capillary refill may indicate problems with cardiac output.

Do the following to evaluate capillary refill:

Step	Action
1	Lift the child's arm or leg slightly above the level of the heart.
2	Press on the skin and release.
3	Count the number of seconds until skin color returns.

It is best to evaluate capillary refill in an environment that is neither hot nor cold. A cold environment may prolong capillary refill time.

Causes of delayed or prolonged capillary refill time (a refill time greater than 2 seconds) include

- Dehydration
- Shock
- Hypothermia

Children with normal capillary refill time may still be in shock. For example, some children with septic shock may have a very rapid (ie, less than 1 second) capillary refill time.

Skin Color and Temperature

Monitor changes in skin color and temperature (as well as capillary refill time) over time to assess a child's response to therapy. Skin color should be consistent over the trunk, arms, and legs. The mucous membranes, nail beds, palms of the hands, and soles of the feet should be pink. Skin temperature should be warm.

When blood flow decreases, the hands and feet are typically affected first. They may become cool, pale, mottled, or cyanotic (bluish or dusky). If the condition worsens, the skin over the arms, legs, and trunk will then become cool with poor color.

Detailed and Advanced Concepts

Consider the temperature of the child's environment when assessing skin color and temperature. If the environment is cool, the child may have cool skin with poor color even though circulation is good. Mottling or pallor with cool skin may be present. Capillary refill may be delayed, particularly in the fingers, toes, hands, and feet.

To assess skin temperature, use the back of your hand, which is more sensitive to temperature changes than the palm. Slide the back of your hand up the child's arm or leg to see if there is a point where the skin temperature changes from cool to warm. Monitor this point between the warm and cool skin over time. Changes will give information about the child's response to intervention. The point of temperature change should move down the limb as the child's condition improves.

Carefully evaluate *pallor*, *mottling*, and *cyanosis*, which may indicate inadequate oxygen delivery to the tissues.

Pallor

Pallor, or paleness, is a lack of normal color in the skin or mucous membranes. Causes of pallor include

- Decreased blood flow to the skin (can be caused by cold, stress, hypovolemic shock)
- Decreased number of red blood cells (anemia)
- Decreased skin pigmentation

Pallor does not necessarily indicate a problem; it can result from lack of sunlight or inherited paleness. However, even if the skin is pale, the mucous membranes should be pink.

> *Look at the mucous membranes, including the lips, lining of the mouth, tongue, and lining of the eyes. If the child has pale mucous membranes or pale palms and soles, look for other signs of shock.*

Pallor is often difficult to detect in a child with dark or thick skin. Family members often can tell you whether a child's color is abnormal. Pallor of the mucous membranes strongly suggests anemia or very poor circulation (shock).

Mottling

Mottling, or mottled skin, is an irregular or patchy discoloration of the skin. When mottling is present, some irregular skin areas are pink, whereas others may appear pale or cyanotic. Mottling may occur as a result of

- Variations in skin coloring
- Cold or cool skin temperature
- Shock (eg, hypovolemia, septic shock)
- Decreased oxygen saturation in the blood (ie, respiratory problems)

Shock and a decrease in oxygen saturation in the blood result in an irregular supply of oxygenated blood to the skin. Severe shock or a severe decrease in the oxygen saturation of the blood may even produce cyanosis in some areas.

Cyanosis

Cyanosis is a bluish discoloration of the skin and mucous membranes. Blood that is fully saturated with oxygen is bright red; blood with less oxygen is dark red, purple, or even blue. Cyanosis may be easier to see in the mucous membranes and nail beds, particularly in children with darker skin. It can also appear on the feet, nose, and ears. Cyanosis may be caused by low blood flow (shock, a circulatory problem) or a low level of oxygen in the blood (eg, a respiratory problem).

If cyanosis is present, it is important to note whether the cyanosis is peripheral or central.

Type of Cyanosis	Location	Possible Cause
Peripheral	Hands and feet	Low blood flow
Central	Mucous membranes	Low oxygen level

In either case, if you see cyanosis, you need to get help.

> *A child who develops central cyanosis typically needs emergency interventions, such as oxygen and support of ventilation.*

Blood Pressure

To measure blood pressure accurately, you must use a properly sized cuff. The cuff bladder should cover about 40% of the circumference of the mid-upper arm. The blood pressure cuff should cover at least 50% to 75% of the length of the upper arm.

Normal Blood Pressures

Table 2 lists normal blood pressure values by age and gender. As with heart rate, there is a wide range of values within the normal range.

Table 2. Normal Blood Pressures by Age

Age	Systolic Blood Pressure (mm Hg)		Diastolic Blood Pressure (mm Hg)	
	Female	Male	Female	Male
Neonate (1 day)	60 to 76	60 to 74	31 to 45	30 to 44
Neonate (4 days)	67 to 83	68 to 84	37 to 53	35 to 53

(continued)

(continued)

Age	Systolic Blood Pressure (mm Hg)		Diastolic Blood Pressure (mm Hg)	
	Female	Male	Female	Male
Infant (1 month)	73 to 91	74 to 94	36 to 56	37 to 55
Infant (3 months)	78 to 100	81 to 103	44 to 64	45 to 65
Infant (6 months)	82 to 102	87 to 105	46 to 66	48 to 68
Infant (1 year)	86 to 104	85 to 103	40 to 58	37 to 56
Child (2 years)	88 to 105	88 to 106	45 to 63	42 to 61
Child (7 years)	96 to 113	97 to 115	57 to 75	57 to 76
Adolescent (15 years)	110 to 127	113 to 131	65 to 83	64 to 83

This table summarizes the range of systolic and diastolic blood pressures according to age and gender from 1 standard deviation below to 1 standard deviation above the mean in the first year of life and from the 50th to 95th percentile (assuming the 50th percentile for height) for children 1 year of age or older.

Blood pressure ranges for neonate and infant (1 to 6 months) are from Gemelli M, Manganaro R, Mamì C, De Luca F. Longitudinal study of blood pressure during the 1st year of life. *Eur J Pediatr.* 1990;149:318-320.

Blood pressure ranges for infant (1 year), child, and adolescent are from National High Blood Pressure Education Program Working Group on High Blood Pressure in Children and Adolescents. *The Fourth Report on the Diagnosis, Evaluation, and Treatment of High Blood Pressure in Children and Adolescents.* Bethesda, MD: National Heart, Lung, and Blood Institute; 2005. NIH publication 05-5267.

Hypotension

Hypotension is defined by the following thresholds of systolic blood pressure (Table 3).

Table 3. Threshold by Age of Systolic Blood Pressure Indicating Hypotension

Age	Systolic Blood Pressure
Term neonates (0 to 28 days)	Less than 60 mm Hg
Infants (1 to 12 months)	Less than 70 mm Hg
Children 1 to 10 years (5th blood pressure percentile)	Less than 70 + (age in years × 2) mm Hg
Children older than 10 years	Less than 90 mm Hg

Note that these blood pressure values overlap with normal blood pressure values for about 5% of healthy children.

Remember that these threshold values are based on studies of normal, resting children. Children with injury and stress will typically have high blood pressure. A blood pressure in the low-normal range may indicate a problem in a seriously ill or injured child. If a child's systolic blood pressure falls 10 mm Hg from baseline, immediately evaluate the child for additional signs of shock.

Detailed and Advanced Concepts	Hypotension in the child is a sign of severe shock. Children in shock can maintain normal blood pressure for some time by increasing the heart rate (tachycardia) and constriction (narrowing) of the blood vessels.
	Hypotension may be a sign of septic shock. In this condition the main problem is excessive dilation (relaxation and enlargement) of the blood vessels.
	A child with a fast heart rate and low blood pressure may develop a *slow* heart rate when his condition worsens. This is a sign of a life-threatening problem. You should get help. Support airway, breathing, and oxygenation. The child will need urgent support of the circulation, such as administration of a fluid bolus.

Other Signs of Circulation

As noted earlier, the child's level of consciousness will help you evaluate blood flow to the brain. See the section "Disability" below for a discussion on evaluating level of consciousness.

Urine output can reflect the blood flow to the kidneys. Normal urine output requires adequate blood flow and hydration. Normal values for urine output are age dependent:

Age	Normal Urine Output
Infants and young children	1.5 to 2 mL/kg per hour
Older children and adolescents	1 mL/kg per hour

Children in shock typically have decreased blood flow to the kidneys and decreased urine output. The initial urine output after insertion of a urinary catheter is not a reliable indicator of the blood flow to the kidneys because much of that urine may have been produced before the onset of symptoms. An increase in the urine output over time is a good indicator of a positive response to therapy.

Disability

D

Evaluate Disability

The disability assessment is a quick evaluation of neurologic function. Clinical signs of brain function are important signs of overall blood flow and oxygen delivery. As you form your initial impression and perform the primary assessment, you should note the child's level of consciousness, muscle tone, and pupil response to light.

A sudden or severe decrease in oxygen delivery in the brain may produce a decreased level of consciousness, loss of muscle tone, and decreased pupil response to light.

Seizures may develop if blood flow to the brain suddenly decreases. Monitor the child for the following signs of decreased oxygen delivery to the brain:

- Confusion
- Irritability
- Lethargy
- Agitation alternating with lethargy

These signs can be subtle and are best detected with repeated observations over time.

> *As a child's level of consciousness decreases, the child will progress from irritability, agitation, or anxiety to decreased responsiveness. These are important clues to the child's clinical condition.*

Evaluate disability by using the following:

- AVPU Pediatric Response Scale
- Response of pupils to light
- Blood glucose test

Repeat the disability evaluation as needed to monitor for changes in the child's neurologic status.

AVPU Pediatric Response Scale

To rapidly evaluate cerebral cortex function, use the AVPU Pediatric Response Scale. This scale is a system for rating a child's level of consciousness. The scale consists of 4 ratings:

Alert	The child is awake, active, and responds appropriately to parents and external stimuli. "Appropriate response" is assessed on the basis of the child's age and the setting or situation.
Voice	The child responds only when you or the parents call the child's name or speak loudly.
Painful	The child responds only to a painful stimulus, such as rubbing the breastbone with your knuckles or pinching a nail bed.
Unresponsive	The child does not respond to any stimulus.

Causes of a decreased level of consciousness in children include

- Decreased blood flow to the brain (eg, severe shock or increased intracranial pressure [ICP])
- Brain injury
- Infection in the brain (eg, encephalitis or meningitis)
- Hypoglycemia (low blood sugar)
- Drug overdose
- Low blood level of oxygen

> *If the child demonstrates a change in level of consciousness or suddenly does not respond to stimulation, call for help. Immediately support airway, breathing, and circulation as needed.*

Response of Pupils to Light

Response of pupils to light is a useful indicator of brainstem function. *If pupil response is abnormal (ie, pupils do not constrict briskly), the child needs advanced life support.*

Normally pupils constrict briskly in response to light and they dilate in a dark environment. Be sure to use a bright light when checking pupil response to light. If the pupils do not constrict in response to direct light stimulus (eg, flashlight directed at the eyes), a brainstem injury may be present. The pupils are generally equal in size; however, slight variations are normal. Irregularities in pupil size or response to light may occur as a result of eye injury or other conditions.

During the disability assessment, record the following for each eye:

- Size of pupils (diameter in millimeters)
- Equality of pupil size (right and left pupils are the same size; right pupil is greater than left pupil; left pupil is greater than right pupil)
- Constriction of pupils to light (ie, the speed of the pupil response to light and the pupil size when constricted)

The acronym PERRL (Pupils Equal, Round, Reactive to Light) describes the normal responses of pupils to light.

Blood Glucose Test

You should monitor the blood glucose level of any seriously ill infant or child. Low blood glucose level may cause altered level of consciousness and other signs. It can cause brain injury if it is not quickly identified and adequately treated. Measure blood glucose level with a point-of-care glucose test.

For more information about the recognition and treatment of hypoglycemia, see Part 8: "Management of Circulatory Emergencies (Shock)."

Exposure

Evaluate Exposure

Exposure is the final component of the primary assessment. When the child is seriously ill or injured, you should measure the child's core temperature. Note any difference in warmth between the trunk and extremities. Identify the presence of fever, which may indicate infection and an early need for antibiotics.

Undress the seriously ill or injured child as necessary to perform a focused physical examination. Remove clothing from one area at a time to carefully observe the child's face, trunk (front and back), extremities, and skin. Keep the child comfortable and warm. If necessary, use blankets and, if available, heating lamps to prevent cold stress or hypothermia.

During this part of the examination, look for rashes or evidence of trauma. You may see petechiae and purpura, which are purple discolorations in the skin that do not blanch with pressure. They are caused by bleeding from capillaries and small vessels in the skin and often represent a serious or life-threatening problem, such as severe infection, septic shock, or a bleeding problem.

Type of Purple Skin Discoloration	Appearance	Possible Problem
Petechiae	Tiny dots	Low platelet count
Purpura	Larger spots	Severe infection or septic shock

Look for injury, bleeding, burns, or unusual marks that might suggest nonaccidental trauma. Some signs of nonaccidental trauma include bruises in different stages of healing or injuries that are inconsistent with the child's history. Another sign is delay from time of injury until medical attention is sought.

If you suspect the child has a head or neck injury, minimize movement of the head and neck. Feel the arms and legs. Note the child's response. If there is obvious tenderness to touch, that area may be injured. You may need to immobilize the arm or leg.

Be Alert for Life-Threatening Conditions

If you detect a life-threatening problem at any time during your assessment, get help. You should also support the child's airway, breathing, and circulation. Signs of a life-threatening condition may include the following:

Airway	Complete or severe airway obstruction
Breathing	Apnea, slow respiratory rate, very fast respiratory rate, very increased or inadequate respiratory effort
Circulation	Absence of palpable pulses, signs of poor perfusion, hypotension, bradycardia
Disability	Unresponsiveness, decreased level of consciousness
Exposure	Significant hypothermia, significant bleeding, petechiae or purpura

Detailed and Advanced Concepts

Immediately begin life-saving interventions and activate emergency response as indicated in your practice setting in the following circumstances:

- If the child has a life-threatening condition
- If you are uncertain or "something feels wrong"

If the child does not have a life-threatening problem, advanced providers may perform the secondary assessment and order diagnostic tests. These are discussed in detail in the *PALS Provider Manual*.

Secondary Assessment

Brief Summary

The secondary assessment consists of a focused medical history obtained by using the SAMPLE mnemonic and a focused physical examination. SAMPLE stands for

- **S**igns and symptoms
- **A**llergies
- **M**edications
- **P**ast medical history
- **L**ast meal
- **E**vents leading to presentation

See the *PALS Provider Manual* for a detailed discussion of the secondary assessment.

Diagnostic Tests

Brief Summary

Diagnostic tests include laboratory, radiographic, and other tests to help find the cause and determine the severity of the child's problem. Tests are performed on the basis of the child's condition. See the *PALS Provider Manual* for more information on specific tests.

Identification of Shock

After "evaluate," the next step in the evaluate-identify-intervene sequence is to identify if the problem is circulatory, respiratory, or both. If the problem is circulatory, the child may be in shock. *Early identification and treatment* of shock are key to improving outcomes in critically ill or injured children. If left untreated, shock can quickly deteriorate to cardiac arrest. Once a child is in cardiac arrest, the chance of survival is low.

Identifying the type and severity of shock will help you prioritize interventions. These interventions are discussed in Part 8: "Management of Circulatory Emergencies (Shock)."

> *If you recognize shock and start therapy immediately, you increase the child's chance for a good outcome.*

Definition of Shock

Shock is a critical condition that results when the tissues do not get as much oxygen as they need. Children in shock often, but not always, have inadequate blood flow. *If signs of poor perfusion are present, the child is in shock, even if the blood pressure is normal.*

Signs of Poor Perfusion
• Tachycardia
• Weak or absent peripheral pulses
• Normal or weak central pulses
• Delayed capillary refill time
• Changes in skin color (pallor, mottling, cyanosis)
• Cool skin
• Decreased level of consciousness
• Decreased urine output

For most children in shock, the amount of blood (blood flow) pumped by the heart is low. Some children in shock, however, have a higher than normal blood flow. High blood flow is often seen in septic shock or in a child with severe anemia. All forms of shock can result in impaired function of vital organs, such as

- The brain: decreased level of consciousness
- The kidneys: low urine output, decreased kidney function

Causes of Shock

Shock can result from several different causes, including

- Inadequate blood volume
- Inappropriate distribution of blood flow
- Impaired pumping of the heart
- Obstructed blood flow

Any problems that cause the tissues to need more oxygen can make shock worse. Such problems include fever, infection, injury, respiratory distress, and pain.

The important point to remember is that, in shock, *tissues are not getting as much oxygen as they need to function properly* because of

- Inadequate oxygen delivery to the tissues
- Increased demand of the tissues for oxygen

When tissues are starved for oxygen, cell and organ damage can occur. This damage may not be reversible. Death from shock may be rapid or may occur later from organ failure.

The treatment goal for shock is to restore adequate blood flow to the tissues. Effective intervention for shock may prevent organ injury. It may also halt the progression to cardiac arrest.

Identify Shock by Type

Identify the types of shock based on the cause:

Type of Shock	Cause of Shock
Hypovolemic shock, including hemorrhage (bleeding)	Inadequate blood volume
Distributive (eg, septic) shock	Inappropriate distribution of blood flow
Cardiogenic shock*	Impaired pumping of the heart
Obstructive shock*	Obstructed blood flow

*Cardiogenic and obstructive shock are included in this manual for your information but are not covered in the PEARS Provider Course. You will not be tested on cardiogenic or obstructive shock in this course. For more information, please see the *PALS Provider Manual.*

A child in shock may have more than one type of shock simultaneously (ie, distributive [eg, septic] and cardiogenic).

Hypovolemic Shock

Causes of Hypovolemic Shock

Hypovolemia (low level of blood volume) is the most common cause of shock in children worldwide. Fluid loss due to diarrhea is the leading cause of hypovolemic shock. In fact, diarrhea and associated dehydration and electrolyte abnormalities are a major worldwide cause of infant death. Causes of hypovolemic shock include

- Diarrhea
- Vomiting
- Hemorrhage (internal or external)
- Inadequate fluid intake
- High urine output (eg, diabetic ketoacidosis)
- Fluid leak into tissues as may occur with septic shock
- Large burns

You must quickly replace the fluid to stabilize the child in hypovolemic shock. To treat shock you may need to give more fluid by IV or intraosseous (IO) infusion than the amount the child lost.

Signs of Hypovolemic Shock

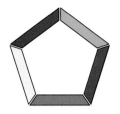

Table 4 outlines typical signs of hypovolemic shock that you might see when evaluating the child during the initial impression and primary assessment.

Table 4. Signs of Hypovolemic Shock

Primary Assessment	Sign
Airway	Typically clear or maintainable unless level of consciousness is significantly impaired
Breathing	Increased respiratory rate without increased effort (quiet tachypnea)

Circulation	• Normal systolic blood pressure or hypotension
	• Signs of poor perfusion
	  – Tachycardia
	  – Weak or absent peripheral pulses
	  – Normal or weak central pulses
	  – Delayed capillary refill time
	  – Changes in skin color (pallor, mottling, cyanosis)
	  – Cool skin
	  – Decreased level of consciousness
	  – Decreased urine output

Disability	Changes in level of consciousness (irritability, agitation, or anxiety to decreased responsiveness)
Exposure	Extremities often cooler than trunk

Distributive Shock

Causes of Distributive Shock

In distributive shock, blood volume is not distributed appropriately. Some tissues receive too much blood flow, and other tissues do not receive enough blood flow.

The most common forms of distributive shock are

- Septic shock
- Anaphylactic shock
- Neurogenic shock (eg, head injury, spinal injury)

In septic, anaphylactic, neurogenic, and other types of distributive shock there is not enough blood flow to some tissues. Blood volume is often decreased as a result of dilation of blood vessels and fluid leaking from the blood vessels. The child must receive IV fluid boluses and drugs to improve heart function and support blood flow. The treatment goal is to increase blood flow to all tissues.

Detailed and Advanced Concepts	The high blood flow and dilation of blood vessels often seen in some children with distributive shock are the opposite of the low blood flow and constriction of blood vessels seen in some other types of shock. In distributive shock, diastolic blood pressure is typically lower than normal. Systolic blood pressure will also fall, especially if you do not give enough IV fluid or you do not give it quickly.

Signs of Distributive Shock

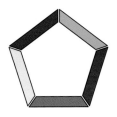

Table 5 outlines typical signs of distributive shock that you might see when evaluating the child during the initial impression and primary assessment. The **bold** text denotes type-specific signs that distinguish distributive shock from other forms of shock.

Table 5. Signs of Distributive Shock

Primary Assessment	Finding
Airway	Typically clear or maintainable unless level of consciousness is significantly impaired; possibly not maintainable if the child has anaphylactic shock
Breathing	• Increased respiratory rate usually without increased respiratory effort • Increased respiratory rate and effort if the child has pneumonia, lung injury, heart failure, pulmonary edema, or anaphylactic shock • Normal breath sounds or crackles
Circulation	Possible signs of poor perfusion *or* • **Warm, flushed skin with brisk capillary refill** • **Peripheral pulses may be bounding** • Normal, low, or high systolic and diastolic blood pressures
Disability	Changes in level of consciousness (agitation, confusion, or decreased responsiveness in late shock)
Exposure	• Fever or hypothermia • Extremities warm or cool • Petechial or purpuric rash (septic shock)

Septic Shock

Causes of Septic Shock

Septic shock is the most common form of distributive shock. It is caused by the body's response to infection. The body's response to infection stimulates the immune system and triggers the release of substances that cause inflammation.

Role of Inflammation in Septic Shock

In the early stages of sepsis, an inflammatory response occurs throughout the body. The illness progresses to septic shock in the late stages. The child's signs may evolve over days or take only hours. The clinical signs and progression vary widely and are caused by the following sequence of events:

- The infectious organism or its byproducts activate inflammation.
- Inflammatory substances, known as cytokines, become active.
- Cytokines cause blood vessels to dilate. Cytokines also cause fluid to leak into the tissues.
- Cytokines and other inflammatory products may also reduce the pumping function of the heart.

Widespread activation of inflammatory substances can lead to organ failure, particularly

- Decreased pumping function of the heart, dilation of blood vessels, and hypotension (shock)
- Severe respiratory distress
- Abnormal clot formation or bleeding
- Decreased production of stress hormone (cortisol)

Signs of Septic Shock   In the early stages signs of septic shock may be difficult to detect. Circulation to the arms and legs may appear to be normal. Because septic shock is triggered by an infection or its byproducts, the child may also have

- Fever or a low temperature for infants younger than 1 year
- Changes in level of consciousness (such as confusion or irritability)
- An elevated or decreased white blood cell count or abnormalities in clotting function
- Petechial or purpuric rash

Treatment Considerations   Because fluid is leaking into the tissues, you should anticipate that the child may develop pulmonary edema (fluid in the lungs) when you give large amounts of IV fluid rapidly. Look for signs of respiratory distress, and be prepared to support the airway, oxygenation, and ventilation. Even if respiratory distress develops, you will still need to give adequate fluid to restore blood flow.

Early recognition and treatment of septic shock are important to good outcome. You should identify signs of shock before hypotension develops. See Part 8: "Management of Circulatory Emergencies (Shock)" for more information.

Anaphylactic Shock

Causes of Anaphylactic Shock   Anaphylactic shock results from a severe reaction to a drug, vaccine, food, toxin, plant, venom, or other antigen. This acute reaction typically starts seconds to minutes after exposure.

In anaphylactic shock the body releases histamine and other inflammatory responses. These substances constrict the airways. They can also dilate the blood vessels and cause fluid leak into the tissues. The child can develop upper airway obstruction from rapid swelling of the tongue and tissues of the upper airway. The fluid leak can produce hypotension. As in septic shock, there is an unbalanced distribution of blood flow, so some tissues do not receive adequate blood flow.

Signs and Symptoms of Anaphylactic Shock

Signs and symptoms of anaphylactic shock may include the following:

Sign	Resulting From
Anxiety or agitation	Low oxygen level
Respiratory distress with stridor, wheezing, or both	Swelling of the tongue and tissues of the upper airway from fluid leak; constriction of airways by inflammatory responses
Hives	Histamine release
Swelling of the face, lips, and tongue	Fluid leak from blood vessels
Hypotension	Dilation of the blood vessels and fluid leaking into the tissues
Tachycardia	Inadequate blood flow to the tissues
Nausea and vomiting	Histamine and other mediator release

Neurogenic Shock

Causes of Neurogenic Shock

Neurogenic shock, including spinal shock, usually results from injury to the cervical spine (neck). The injury disrupts the nerve supply to the blood vessels and the heart. The sudden loss of nervous system signals to smooth muscle in the vessel walls results in dilation of the blood vessels.

Signs of Neurogenic Shock

Primary signs of neurogenic shock are

- Hypotension with a low diastolic blood pressure
- Normal heart rate or bradycardia

Unlike other forms of shock with low or normal blood pressure, *in neurogenic shock the heart rate is not fast; it may even be slower than normal*. This distinguishes neurogenic shock from the other forms of distributive shock.

The spine injury that causes spinal shock also injures the nerves to the skeletal muscles. You will see other signs of a spinal injury (eg, loss of movement or sensation).

It is important to understand the difference between hypovolemic shock with hypotension and neurogenic shock.

Hypovolemic Shock	Neurogenic Shock
Hypotension accompanied by tachycardia	Hypotension accompanied by a normal heart rate or bradycardia

Cardiogenic Shock

Causes of Cardiogenic Shock

A child in cardiogenic shock has poor circulation resulting from decreased pumping function of the heart. This can be caused by pump failure (poor contractility), congenital heart disease, or rhythm abnormalities.

Common causes of cardiogenic shock include

- Abnormality of pumping function
- Injury to the heart (eg, trauma)
- Inflammation of the heart muscle
- Sepsis
- Poisoning or drug toxicity
- Congenital or genetic heart disease
- Abnormal heart rhythm (arrhythmias)

Signs of Cardiogenic Shock

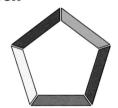

Table 6 outlines typical signs of cardiogenic shock that you might see during the initial impression and primary assessments of the child. The **bold** text denotes type-specific signs that distinguish cardiogenic shock from other forms of shock.

Table 6. Signs of Cardiogenic Shock

Primary Assessment	Finding
Airway	Typically clear or maintainable unless level of consciousness is significantly impaired
Breathing	• Fast respiratory rate • **Increased respiratory effort (retractions, nasal flaring) resulting from pulmonary edema**
Circulation	• Tachycardia • Normal or low blood pressure • Signs of poor perfusion • **Signs of congestive heart failure (eg, pulmonary edema, enlarged liver, distended neck veins)** • **Cyanosis (may or may not be present)**
Disability	Change in level of consciousness (irritability, agitation, or anxiety early, decreased responsiveness later)
Exposure	Extremities often cooler than trunk

Reassessment of a Child in Cardiogenic Shock

In cardiogenic shock, oxygen saturation may be low if lung tissue disease or a cyanotic congenital heart defect is also present.

> A child with cardiogenic shock usually has a fast respiratory rate with increased respiratory effort. By comparison, a child in hypovolemic shock usually has a fast respiratory rate but usually **without** increased respiratory effort.

If a child has *cardiogenic* shock, you should not give large or rapid fluid boluses. The boluses can worsen heart function and increase fluid in the lungs. Remember the following:

- Give small isotonic fluid boluses (5 to 10 mL/kg).
- Give fluid boluses over longer periods of time (ie, 10 to 20 minutes instead of 5 to 10 minutes).
- Monitor the child closely during fluid infusion.

Infants and children with cardiogenic shock often require drug therapy to improve heart function and blood flow. In addition, treatment includes methods to decrease oxygen needs, such as support of respiratory function (eg, mechanical ventilation) and treating fever.

Obstructive Shock

Causes and Types of Obstructive Shock

Obstructive shock is caused by a block in blood flow pathways. Causes include the following:

Cause	Mechanism of Obstruction
Cardiac tamponade	Accumulation of fluid in the sac around the heart
Tension pneumothorax	Accumulation of air between the lung and the chest wall (the lung collapses)
Certain heart defects that require the ductus arteriosus (which normally closes after birth) to stay open	Obstruction of normal blood flow from the heart into the pulmonary artery or into the aorta
Pulmonary embolism	Blood clot to the lungs that obstructs blood flow

The obstruction to blood flow results in decreased blood flow to the tissues. As the condition progresses, increased respiratory effort, cyanosis, and signs of poor circulation become more apparent.

Importance of Rapid Identification

The treatment of obstructive shock is cause specific. Immediate identification and correction of the underlying cause of the obstruction can be lifesaving.

> *If you think the child has obstructive shock, get help immediately. Without immediate advanced treatment, children with obstructive shock often progress rapidly to cardiac arrest.*

Obstructive shock is uncommon in children but may be seen in children with congenital heart disease, severe respiratory disease, or trauma. For more information, see the *PALS Provider Manual*.

Identify Shock by Severity (Effect on Blood Pressure)

The severity of shock is categorized by the effect on the child's systolic blood pressure.

Compensated shock	Signs of poor perfusion and normal systolic blood pressure
Hypotensive* shock	Signs of poor perfusion and low systolic blood pressure (hypotension)

*Hypotensive shock was previously referred to as "decompensated" shock.

Identifying the severity of shock as compensated or hypotensive provides a simple way to recognize when very rapid interventions are needed.

Identifying the Severity of Shock

Hypotensive shock is easy to recognize when you measure blood pressure. Compensated shock may be more difficult to identify. The signs and symptoms of shock are affected by the

- Type of shock
- Cause of shock

Remember, severe shock may occur with normal or low blood pressure. In some cases, children with low systolic blood pressure will still have enough blood flow to meet tissue demand. On the other hand, some children with normal blood pressure may be in severe shock. These children will have other symptoms such as absent peripheral pulses and decreased level of consciousness.

You should **not** rely on a blood pressure reading alone to categorize shock severity. Make decisions on the basis of the entire assessment. Use your initial impression evaluation of consciousness, breathing, and color. Then use your primary assessment evaluation of heart rate, peripheral and central pulses, capillary refill time, and skin color and temperature. Remember these important points:

- Automated blood pressure devices are accurate only when the child has adequate circulation to the arms and legs. If you cannot palpate peripheral pulses and the arms and legs are cool with delayed capillary refill, an automated blood pressure reading may not be reliable.
- Infants and children with compensated shock may be critically ill with severe shock despite a normal systolic blood pressure.

Note that in compensated shock, the *systolic* pressure is normal, but the *diastolic* pressure may be abnormal (ie, low or high).

Compensated Shock

If the child has a normal systolic blood pressure but has signs of poor perfusion, the child is in compensated shock. In this stage of shock, the body is still able to maintain adequate blood pressure and blood flow to the brain and the heart. The body typically reduces blood flow to organs such as the skin and kidneys and redirects it to the brain and heart. These changes in blood flow produce some of the signs of shock. The signs vary according to the type and severity of shock.

During your assessment of a seriously ill or injured child, look for these signs of poor perfusion, which indicate the child is in shock (Table 7).

Table 7. Signs of Poor Perfusion

Area	Sign
Heart	Tachycardia
Pulses	Weak or absent peripheral pulses
	Normal or weak central pulses
Skin	Delayed capillary refill time (in septic shock capillary refill may be delayed or very rapid)
	Changes in skin color (pallor, mottling, cyanosis)
	Cool skin (in septic shock skin may be cold or warm)
Brain	Decreased level of consciousness (irritability, agitation, or anxiety to decreased responsiveness)
Kidney	Decreased urine output

Signs specific to the cause of shock are discussed earlier in this Part.

Hypotensive Shock

The child has hypotensive shock if the following are present:

- Systolic hypotension
- Signs of poor perfusion

Hypotension develops when attempts to maintain systolic blood pressure and blood flow are no longer effective. One key clinical sign that a child's condition is getting worse is a decrease in level of consciousness. This occurs when there is not enough blood flow to the brain. The child's level of consciousness may progress from irritability, agitation, or anxiety to decreased responsiveness. Hypotension is a late finding in most types of shock. Unless rapidly corrected, it may be a sign that shock cannot be reversed, and cardiac arrest may occur soon.

Blood Pressure Formulas

Use the following formulas to evaluate blood pressure and to identify hypotension:

Age (years)	Range	Formula
1 to 10	Estimate of typical systolic blood pressure (50th percentile)	90 + (age in years × 2) mm Hg
1 to 10	Threshold of systolic blood pressure indicating hypotension	Less than 70 + (age in years × 2) mm Hg
Older than 10	Threshold of systolic blood pressure indicating hypotension	Less than 90 mm Hg

See Table 3: Threshold by Age of Systolic Blood Pressure Indicating Hypotension in Part 7.

Progression of Shock

Watch closely for signs that the child's condition is getting worse. If untreated, a child in shock will likely progress from compensated shock to hypotensive shock and then to cardiac arrest. Warning signs include

- Absence of peripheral pulses
- Decrease in level of consciousness/responsiveness

Bradycardia and weak-to-absent central pulses typically indicate severe problems and risk of progression to cardiac arrest.

Accelerating Process

It may take hours for the child in compensated shock to progress to hypotensive shock. It may take only minutes for the child in hypotensive shock to progress to cardiac arrest. The progression from compensated shock to hypotensive shock and then to cardiac arrest is typically an *accelerating process.*

Compensated Shock

Possibly hours

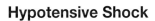

Hypotensive Shock

Potentially minutes

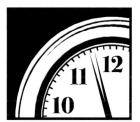

Cardiac Arrest

Act quickly to treat compensated shock. Your rapid interventions may prevent progression to hypotensive shock and cardiac arrest.

Part 8

Management of Circulatory Emergencies (Shock)

Overview

Once you identify shock in a seriously ill or injured child, immediate intervention can greatly improve outcome.

This Part discusses goals of shock management and interventions for a child in shock. It also includes information on fluid therapy and the importance of monitoring blood glucose.

Learning Objectives

After completing this Part you should be able to

- Describe the general goals of shock management
- Summarize the initial priorities for stabilizing a child in shock
- Describe principles of effective IV fluid bolus therapy for shock
- Explain how effective shock therapy depends on identifying the type and severity of shock
- State the volume and rate of fluid administration for shock

Preparation for the Course

During the PEARS Course you will actively participate in instructor-led shock case discussions. Study this part so that you will know appropriate interventions for a child in shock.

Goals of Shock Management

The goals in management of shock are to

- Improve oxygen content of the blood
- Improve blood flow to the tissues
- Reduce tissue demand for oxygen
- Support organ function
- Prevent cardiac arrest

Immediate intervention for a child in shock may be lifesaving. The more time that passes between the event that caused the shock and the start of treatment, the worse the outcome will be. If a child in shock progresses to cardiac arrest, the chance of survival is generally poor.

Warning Signs

You must be alert to signs that a seriously ill or injured child is getting worse. Warning signs that a child in shock is getting worse include

- Increasing tachycardia
- Absent peripheral pulses
- Weakening central pulses
- Cold hands and feet with very prolonged capillary refill
- Decreased level of consciousness
- Hypotension (late finding)

Once hypotension develops, organ damage may occur even if the child does not develop cardiac arrest.

> *Early recognition of compensated shock is critical to effective intervention and good outcome.*

Initial Management of Shock

Initial management of a child in shock may include the interventions summarized in Table 2 later in this Part. Your quick actions may be lifesaving for a child in shock. The actions you take will be based on your scope of practice and local protocols.

> *If you identify the signs of shock, you should get help or seek expert consultation.*

General management of shock consists of the following:

- Getting help
- Positioning of the child
- Oxygen administration
- Ventilation support
- Vascular access
- IV fluid therapy
- Monitoring
- Frequent evaluation

Note that many of these interventions may be carried out at the same time.

Getting Help

Remember that for some types of shock, lifesaving interventions may be required that are beyond your scope of practice. Sometimes the most important intervention for a child in shock is getting help. This includes calling a resuscitation team, activating emergency response, or alerting more advanced providers.

Positioning of the Child	Positioning is important for a child in shock.

- Open and maintain the airway. Be prepared to support the airway if necessary.
- Place a hypotensive child in the supine position. Make sure that breathing is not compromised.

Oxygen Administration

Be sure that the child has an open airway. Prepare to support the airway if necessary. Give humidified high-flow oxygen to all children in shock.

Ventilation Support

Assess respiratory rate and effort. Be prepared to support ventilation with a bag-mask device as needed.

Vascular Access

Once you support airway and breathing, the next priority is to gain vascular access. Vascular access is needed for fluid therapy and drug administration. For children in compensated shock, venous access is preferred if it can be obtained rapidly. If not, IO access should be established. IO access is a type of vascular access used in emergencies. For children in hypotensive shock, immediate vascular access is critical.

> *For children in hypotensive shock, immediate vascular access is needed. Be prepared to establish IO access if IV access can't be obtained quickly.*

IV Fluid Therapy

Once vascular access is established, give fluid boluses immediately.

> *Give isotonic crystalloid* (normal saline [NS] or lactated Ringer's [LR]) as a 20 mL/kg bolus over 5 to 20 minutes to restore blood flow and blood pressure. Multiple boluses are often necessary. Remember that if you suspect that the pumping function of the heart is poor, you should give smaller fluid boluses (about 5 to 10 mL/kg) over a longer period of time (about 10 to 20 minutes).*
>
> **See "Isotonic Crystalloid Solutions" later in this Part.*

As you give the fluid bolus, monitor for

- Development or worsening of signs of respiratory distress (may indicate the presence of fluid in the lungs)
- Decrease in oxygen saturation
- Decreased perfusion or weak pulses

Be prepared to support oxygenation and ventilation if necessary.

Monitoring

Assess the effectiveness of fluid resuscitation by frequent or continuous monitoring (Table 1).

Table 1. Monitoring in Circulatory Emergencies

Frequently or Continuously Monitor	Expected Normal Finding
Oxygen saturation with pulse oximetry	94% or higher when breathing room air
Heart rate	See Table 1 in Part 7
Peripheral pulses	No longer weak or bounding
Capillary refill	Less than 2 seconds
Skin color and temperature	Normal skin color and mucous membranes
Blood pressure	See Table 2 in Part 7
Level of consciousness	Awake and responds appropriately
Ongoing fluid losses	Bleeding and diarrhea controlled
Urine output	*Infants and young children* Greater than 1.5 to 2 mL/kg per hour *Older children and adolescents* Greater than 1 mL/kg per hour

Frequent Evaluation

Frequently evaluate the child's breathing, circulation, and level of consciousness to

- Evaluate trends in the child's condition
- Determine response to therapy
- Plan the next interventions

A child's condition can change rapidly. Frequent evaluation will help you identify when interventions are needed. Reassess frequently until the child's condition is stable or the child is transferred to another level of care.

> *The condition of a child in shock is dynamic. Monitor the child continuously and evaluate frequently. This will help identify trends in the child's condition and the child's response to interventions.*

Summary: General Management

Table 2 summarizes the general management of shock discussed in this section.

> *Remember to get help or seek expert consultation when caring for an infant or child with signs of shock.*

Table 2. Fundamentals of Shock Management

Get help
Position the child • Stable: allow to remain with caregiver • Unstable: if hypotensive, place child on her back unless breathing is compromised
Give high-flow oxygen
Support airway and ventilation as needed
Ensure vascular (IV/IO) access • Consider IO access early (according to scope of practice)
Begin IV/IO fluid bolus therapy for shock • Give bolus (20 mL/kg) of isotonic crystalloid over 5 to 20 minutes. • Give a smaller volume (5 to 10 mL/kg) over 10 to 20 minutes if poor heart function is present or suspected.
Monitor • Oxygen saturation with pulse oximetry • Heart rate • Peripheral pulses • Capillary refill time • Skin color and temperature • Blood pressure • Urine output • Level of consciousness • Blood glucose
Perform frequent reassessments • Evaluate trends • Identify response to therapy

IV Fluid Therapy for Shock

Intervention for shock includes IV or IO fluid therapy. The primary goal of fluid therapy is to restore adequate blood flow to the tissues. The rate and volume of fluid therapy are determined by the type and severity of the child's shock. Rapid fluid therapy is used to treat hypovolemic and distributive shock. Other types of shock and conditions require adjustment of rate and volume.

Either isotonic crystalloid or colloid solutions may be used for fluid therapy. Blood and blood products are used for replacement of blood loss or correction of some disorders of blood clotting. However, they are generally not the first choice for fluid replacement in children with shock.

Remember to get help if you identify shock and need to give a fluid bolus.

Isotonic Crystalloid Solutions

For a child in shock, the preferred initial fluid for volume replacement is an isotonic crystalloid solution such as

- Normal saline
- Lactated Ringer's

These fluids are inexpensive and readily available. They also have few complications. To treat hypovolemic shock, you will likely have to give several fluid boluses.

Rapid infusion of a large volume of fluid is usually well tolerated by a healthy child. A large volume of fluid, however, should not be used in the critically ill child with underlying cardiac or renal disease.

Do not use fluid containing dextrose (glucose) as a bolus for shock; the child may develop hyperglycemia. This can result in increased urine output and make hypovolemia and shock worse. Electrolyte imbalances can also develop.

Rate and Volume of Fluid Therapy for Shock

Start a fluid bolus for a child in shock. A typical fluid bolus is 20 mL/kg of isotonic crystalloid. Give the fluid bolus over 5 to 20 minutes, depending on the type of shock. If you do not know the child's weight, use a color-coded length-based resuscitation tape to quickly estimate it.

Determine the correct volume of isotonic fluid and rate of delivery based on type of shock:

Type of Shock	Volume of Fluid	Rate of Delivery
• Hypovolemic shock • Distributive shock	20 mL/kg	*Give fluid bolus more rapidly* (ie, over 5 to 10 minutes)
• Cardiogenic shock (poor pumping function of the heart)	5 to 10 mL/kg (ie, smaller volume of fluid)	*Give fluid bolus more slowly* (ie, over 10 to 20 minutes)

Reevaluate the child after each fluid bolus and repeat fluid bolus as needed. Adjust fluid therapy for conditions such as shock associated with diabetic ketoacidosis, burns, and some poisonings. See the *PALS Provider Manual* for more information.

Rapid Fluid Delivery

The equipment used for routine IV pediatric fluid administration cannot deliver fluid boluses as rapidly as needed for a child in shock. The following are some ways to help deliver fluid quickly:

- Use a large-diameter catheter, especially for blood or colloid
- Place an inline, 3-way stopcock in the IV tubing system
- Use a 35-mL to 60-mL syringe attached to a 3-way stopcock to give fluids rapidly
- Use a pressure bag
- Consider rapid infusion devices

Note: A rapid infusion rate with an IV infusion pump (eg, a rate of 999 mL/h) does not provide an adequate fluid bolus delivery rate for a child weighing greater than 20 kg. For example, a 50-kg child with septic shock should ideally receive 1 liter of crystalloid in 10 minutes. It would take 1 hour to deliver this amount of fluid with an infusion pump set to administer 999 mL/h. This rate is too slow for fluid bolus delivery for a child in shock.

Frequent Evaluation

Frequently evaluate the child during fluid resuscitation. Monitor to

- Assess the response to therapy after each fluid bolus
- Determine the need for additional fluid boluses
- Assess for increased respiratory effort or other signs of fluid in the lungs during and after each IV fluid bolus

Monitor the child's condition for improvement (Table 1). If the child's condition gets worse after fluid therapy, you should consider that other types of shock may be present, such as cardiogenic or obstructive shock. Increased work of breathing may indicate development of pulmonary edema (fluid in the lungs) and the need for support of ventilation.

Glucose

It is important to monitor blood glucose concentration in a child with signs of shock. Hypoglycemia is a common finding in critically ill children. It can result in brain injury if it is not recognized and effectively treated. Glucose is also necessary for normal heart function, particularly in young infants.

Glucose Monitoring

Measure blood glucose concentration in *all* infants and children with decreased level of consciousness, shock, or severe respiratory distress. Glucose can be measured with a point-of-care device or by laboratory analysis.

You should not use fluids containing glucose for fluid bolus therapy. However, it may be necessary to give glucose if hypoglycemia is documented or strongly suspected. Small infants and chronically ill children have limited stores of glycogen (the form in which glucose is stored in the body). During episodes of shock these stores may be rapidly depleted, resulting in hypoglycemia. Infants receiving non–glucose-containing IV fluids are at increased risk for developing hypoglycemia.

> *If point-of-care testing is available, perform a rapid glucose test for all critically ill or injured children to evaluate for the presence of hypoglycemia. If hypoglycemia is present, you should intervene quickly and get help.*

How to Perform a Point-of-Care Glucose Test

Although you will not perform a rapid point-of-care (bedside) glucose test during the course, it is important to remember that all critically ill or injured children should have a glucose test to rule out hypoglycemia. Hypoglycemia can be a cause of shock or decreased level of consciousness.

The following steps are a general guide for performing a rapid bedside glucose test. Modify these steps as appropriate, based on the device used and local protocols.

Step	Action
1	Clean the puncture site.
2	Insert a fresh lancet into the lancet device if required.
3	Prepare the blood glucose meter and test strip. (This step will vary according to manufacturer.)

(continued)

(continued)

Step	Action
4	Use the lancet to obtain a small drop of blood from the puncture site.
5	Put the drop of blood on the test strip and insert it into the blood glucose meter.
6	The meter will display the results.
7	Dispose of the used lancet in an approved container.

Diagnosis of Hypoglycemia

Hypoglycemia may be difficult to identify by the child's appearance. Some infants and children may have few symptoms of hypoglycemia. Others may have nonspecific signs. Nonspecific signs are poor perfusion, tachycardia, hypotension, sweating, irritability or lethargy, and hypothermia. These may also indicate other problems or conditions, such as low oxygen saturation and shock.

In addition to the measured glucose concentration thresholds listed below, symptomatic hypoglycemia is defined by the presence of clinical signs such as

- Tachycardia
- Sweating
- Altered level of consciousness (agitation, lethargy, or seizures)

Although specific values are not applicable to every patient, the following lowest acceptable glucose concentrations can be used to define hypoglycemia:

Age	Consensus Definition of Hypoglycemia
Preterm neonates **Term neonates**	Less than 45 mg/dL
Infants **Children** **Adolescents**	Less than 60 mg/dL

The definition for hypoglycemia listed in the table is based on samples from healthy fasting infants and children. The glucose concentration may be higher in children who are stressed, critically ill, or injured.

Management of Hypoglycemia

The following are recommendations for managing hypoglycemia:

If...	Intervene by Administering...
The glucose concentration is low in a responsive child	Oral glucose (eg, juice or other glucose-containing fluid) as long as the child is not in shock
The glucose concentration is low and the child is unresponsive or in shock	IV/IO dextrose (dextrose is the same as glucose)

If hypoglycemia is treated with IV dextrose (0.5 to 1 g/kg), administer one of the following:

- $D_{25}W$ (25% dextrose in water): 2 to 4 mL/kg
- $D_{10}W$ (10% dextrose in water): 5 to 10 mL/kg

Evaluate the blood glucose concentration with point-of-care testing after administration of dextrose.

> *Remember to get help if you identify a low glucose concentration.*

Equipment and Procedures for Management of Circulatory Emergencies

Preparation for the Course

The following skills may be demonstrated during the PEARS Provider Course:

Topic	Page
Cardiac Monitoring	111
Fluid Resuscitation	112
Color-Coded Length-Based Resuscitation Tape	113
Epinephrine Autoinjector	114

Cardiac Monitoring

Cardiac Monitoring Procedure

Follow these steps to connect a cardiac monitor. Modify the sequence for your specific device.

Step	Action
1	**Power on the monitor.**
2	**Attach ECG leads to the child** (Figure 1): • White lead—to right shoulder • Red lead—to left flank or abdomen • Ground (black, green, brown) lead—to left shoulder **Figure 1.** Placement of leads for ECG monitoring.
3	**Adjust the device to manual ECG monitoring mode** to display ECG in standard limb leads (I, II, III).
4	**Visually check the monitor screen and assess heart rate.**

Fluid Resuscitation

Preparation for the Course

During the case discussions and in your clinical practice, you will need to recognize a child who needs urgent vascular access for fluid resuscitation. You should know the type of fluid bolus to administer to a patient in shock; isotonic crystalloid should be used for initial resuscitation (see "Initial Management of Shock" earlier in this Part). You should also know how to give a fluid bolus.

How to Give a Fluid Bolus With a Syringe and 3-Way Stopcock

Microdrip (60 drops per milliliter) IV systems do not deliver fluid boluses as rapidly as needed for a child in shock. You should know the technique for giving a fluid bolus correctly by using a syringe and 3-way stopcock.

Follow these steps to give a fluid bolus with a syringe and 3-way stopcock.

Step	Action
1	Establish IV/IO access if it is not already in place. Check to be sure that access is patent.
2	Connect a bag of isotonic crystalloid with a 3-way stopcock to the IV/IO access. Join the 3-way stopcock to the existing IV/IO tubing, between the T connector and IV tubing. (When no stopcock is available, attach only a syringe to the injection port.)
3	Attach a large syringe to the stopcock. (If no stopcock is available, you can insert a syringe at an injection port.)
4	To draw up the IV fluid into the syringe: • Turn the stopcock *off* to the child and *open* between the syringe and the bag of isotonic crystalloid. • Pull back on the syringe plunger, filling the syringe with the desired amount of IV fluid. • Turn the stopcock *off* to fluid and *open* between the syringe and the child.
5	To rapidly infuse a fluid bolus: • Be sure that the stopcock is *open* between the child and the syringe and *closed* to the bag of isotonic crystalloid. • Push the syringe plunger, causing the fluid to flow through the tubing into the child. After the bolus is delivered, turn the stopcock *open* between the child and the IV fluid bag (and *off* to the syringe). Reset the IV infusion rate as ordered.

Reassess and reconfirm indications for additional fluid boluses. Repeat this technique for rapid infusion of subsequent boluses as indicated.

Color-Coded Length-Based Resuscitation Tape

Preparation for the Course

During the course you may be asked to use a color-coded length-based resuscitation tape (Table 1). This tape (or similar resource) is often used during an emergency to select the correct sizes of resuscitation equipment and supplies and to determine the child's weight (if not known) for calculating drug doses.

Table 1. Color-Coded Length-Based Resuscitation Tape

Equipment	GRAY* 3-5 kg	PINK Small Infant 6-7 kg	RED Infant 8-9 kg	PURPLE Toddler 10-11 kg	YELLOW Small Child 12-14 kg	WHITE Child 15-18 kg	BLUE Child 19-23 kg	ORANGE Large Child 24-29 kg	GREEN Adult 30-36 kg
Resuscitation bag		Infant/child	Infant/child	Child	Child	Child	Child	Child	Adult
Oxygen mask (NRB)		Pediatric	Pediatric	Pediatric	Pediatric	Pediatric	Pediatric	Pediatric	Pediatric/adult
Oral airway (mm)		50	50	60	60	60	70	80	80
Laryngoscope blade (size)		1 Straight	1 Straight	1 Straight	2 Straight	2 Straight	2 Straight or curved	2 Straight or curved	3 Straight or curved
ET tube (mm)†		3.5 Uncuffed 3.0 Cuffed	3.5 Uncuffed 3.0 Cuffed	4.0 Uncuffed 3.5 Cuffed	4.5 Uncuffed 4.0 Cuffed	5.0 Uncuffed 4.5 Cuffed	5.5 Uncuffed 5.0 Cuffed	6.0 Cuffed	6.5 Cuffed
ET tube insertion length (cm)	3 kg 9-9.5 4 kg 9.5-10 5 kg 10-10.5	10.5-11	10.5-11	11-12	13.5	14-15	16.5	17-18	18.5-19.5
Suction catheter (F)		8	8	10	10	10	10	10	10-12
BP cuff	Neonatal #5/infant	Infant/child	Infant/child	Child	Child	Child	Child	Child	Small adult
IV catheter (ga)		22-24	22-24	20-24	18-22	18-22	18-20	18-20	16-20
IO (ga)		18/15	18/15	15	15	15	15	15	15
NG tube (F)		5-8	5-8	8-10	10	10	12-14	14-18	16-18
Urinary catheter (F)	5	8	8	8-10	10	10-12	10-12	12	12
Chest tube (F)		10-12	10-12	16-20	20-24	20-24	24-32	28-32	32-38

Abbreviations: BP, blood pressure; ET, endotracheal; F, French; IO, intraosseous; IV, intravenous; NG, nasogastric; NRB, nonrebreathing.

*For Gray column, use Pink or Red equipment sizes if no size is listed.

†Per 2010 AHA Guidelines, in the hospital cuffed or uncuffed tubes may be used (see below for sizing of cuffed tubes).

Adapted from Broselow™ Pediatric Emergency Tape. Distributed by Armstrong Medical Industries, Lincolnshire, IL. Copyright 2007 Vital Signs, Inc. All rights reserved.

Epinephrine Autoinjector

Preparation for the Course

You should know the correct technique for using an epinephrine autoinjector.

Correct Technique

Before using the epinephrine autoinjector, quickly examine it to make sure it is safe to use. Do not use it if the

- Solution is discolored
- Clear window on the autoinjector is red

Follow these steps to correctly use an epinephrine autoinjector:

Step	Action
1	Remove the epinephrine autoinjector from the package.
2	Take off the safety cap. Follow the instructions printed on the package.
3	Hold the barrel of the autoinjector in your fist. Do not touch either end of the autoinjector because the needle comes out of one end.
4	Push the end with the needle hard against the side of the child's thigh, about halfway between the hip and knee. You can give the injection through clothes or on bare skin.
5	Hold the autoinjector in place for about 10 seconds.
6	Remove the needle by pulling the pen straight out.

Shock Case Discussions

Shock Case Discussions (Shock Cases 1-2)

During the course you will watch short videos* of seriously ill or injured children in shock. Your instructor will lead the group in a discussion of the PEARS Systematic Approach for each case. These discussions will follow the format outlined below.

*To help improve your assessment skills, the PEARS Course includes videos of actual children with medical problems that you may encounter. These videos may be disturbing to some viewers. In some cases videos were looped or edited to provide you with adequate assessment time and to emphasize key teaching points.

At no time was medical care delayed for the purpose of obtaining video footage. All of these children received timely and appropriate medical care, mainly in children's hospitals. Consent was obtained before any video recording.

Initial Impression

Remember that the initial impression is your first quick (in a few seconds) "from the doorway" observation of the following:

Consciousness	Level of consciousness (eg, unresponsive, irritable, alert)
Breathing	Increased work of breathing, absent or decreased respiratory effort, or abnormal sounds heard without a stethoscope
Color	Abnormal skin color, such as pallor, mottling, or cyanosis

The purpose is to quickly identify a life-threatening problem.

Unresponsive or Responsive?

Is the child unresponsive with no breathing or only gasping? If so, provide emergency treatment and call for help.

If the child is responsive, continue the evaluate-identify-intervene sequence.

Continue the Evaluate-Identify-Intervene Sequence

Use the **evaluate-identify-intervene** sequence when caring for a seriously ill or injured child.

- *Evaluate* the child to gather information about the child's condition or status.
- *Identify* any problem by type and severity.
- *Intervene* with appropriate actions to treat the problem.

Then repeat the sequence; this process is ongoing.

Evaluate

Evaluate by using the primary assessment. In the respiratory cases you only evaluated A and B. For the circulatory cases you will need to evaluate ABCDE.

Please refer to the PEARS Systematic Approach Summary on your PEARS Pocket Reference Card or in the Appendix.

Airway

Clear	Maintainable	Not maintainable

Breathing

Respiratory Rate and Pattern	Respiratory Effort		Chest Expansion and Air Movement	Abnormal Lung and Airway Sounds		Oxygen Saturation by Pulse Oximetry
Normal	Normal	Inadequate	Normal	Stridor	Gurgling	Normal oxygen saturation (≥94%)
Irregular	Increased	• Apnea	Decreased	Snoring	Wheezing	
Fast	• Nasal flaring	• Weak cry or cough	Unequal	Barking cough	Crackles	Hypoxemia (<94%)
Slow	• Retractions		Prolonged expiration		Unequal	
Apnea	• Head bobbing			Hoarseness		
	• Seesaw respirations			Grunting		

Circulation

Heart Rate	Pulses		Capillary Refill Time	Skin Color and Temperature		Blood Pressure
	Central	*Peripheral*				
Normal	Normal	Normal	Normal: ≤2 seconds	Pallor	Warm skin	Normal
Fast (tachycardia)	Weak	Weak	Delayed: >2 seconds	Mottling	Cool skin	Hypotensive
Slow (bradycardia)	Absent	Absent		Cyanosis		

Disability

AVPU Pediatric Response Scale				Pupil Size; Reaction to Light		Blood Glucose	
Alert	Responds to **V**oice	Responds to **P**ain	**U**nresponsive	Normal	Abnormal	Normal	Low

Exposure

Temperature			Skin	
Normal	High	Low	Rash (eg, purpura)	Trauma (eg, injury, bleeding)

Identify by Type and Severity

Identify	*Identify the child's problem as respiratory, circulatory, or both. Determine the type and severity of the problem(s). The table below lists common clinical signs that typically correlate with a specific type of problem and its severity.*

	Type	**Severity**
Respiratory	• Upper airway obstruction • Lower airway obstruction • Lung tissue disease • Disordered control of breathing	• Mild respiratory distress • Severe respiratory distress
Circulatory	• Hypovolemic shock • Distributive (eg, septic, anaphylactic) shock • Obstructive shock • Cardiogenic shock	• Compensated shock • Hypotensive shock
Cardiac Arrest		

Identifying Circulatory Emergencies (Shock)		
• Tachycardia • Weak or absent peripheral pulses • Normal or weak central pulses • Delayed capillary refill time	• Changes in skin color (pallor, mottling, cyanosis) • Cool skin • Decreased level of consciousness • Decreased urine output	**Signs of poor perfusion**
Signs	**Type of Problem**	**Severity**
• Signs of poor perfusion (see above)	**Hypovolemic shock**	**Compensated shock** • Signs of poor perfusion and normal systolic blood pressure **Hypotensive shock** • Signs of poor perfusion and low systolic blood pressure (hypotension)
• Possible signs of poor perfusion (see above) *or* • Warm, flushed skin with brisk capillary refill • Peripheral pulses may be bounding • Possible crackles • Possible petechial or purpuric rash (septic shock)	**Distributive shock**	

Intervene

For a quick reference on management of shock, see the Management of Shock Flowchart on your PEARS Pocket Reference Card or in the Appendix.

Management of Shock Flowchart

General Management for All Patients
• Get help
• Position the child
• Give high-flow oxygen
• Support airway and ventilation as needed
• Ensure vascular (IV/IO) access
• Begin IV/IO fluid bolus therapy for shock
• Monitor oxygen saturation, heart rate, peripheral pulses, capillary refill, skin color and temperature, blood pressure, urine output, level of consciousness, blood glucose
• Perform frequent reassessments
Hypovolemic Shock
• 20 mL/kg NS/LR bolus (repeat as needed)
• Control external bleeding (if present)
Distributive (eg, Septic) Shock
• 20 mL/kg NS/LR bolus (repeat as needed)

For more details, see Part 8: "Management of Circulatory Emergencies (Shock)."

Case 1 Notes

Case 2 Notes

Part **10**

BLS Competency Testing

BLS Skills Testing

Testing Requirements

You must pass 2 BLS tests as one of the requirements to receive an American Heart Association (AHA) PEARS Provider course completion card.

BLS Skills Testing Requirements
• Pass 1- and 2-Rescuer Child BLS With AED Skills Test
• Pass 1- and 2-Rescuer Infant BLS Skills Test

BLS Skills Testing Sheets

The 1- and 2-Rescuer Child BLS With AED Skills Testing Sheet and the 1- and 2-Rescuer Infant BLS Skills Testing Sheet provide detailed descriptions of the CPR skills that you will be expected to perform. Your instructor will evaluate your CPR skills during the skills test on the basis of these descriptions.

If you perform a specific skill exactly as described in the critical performance criteria details, the instructor will check that specific skill as "passing." If you do not perform a specific skill exactly as it is described, the skill will not be checked off, and you will require remediation in that skill.

Study the BLS skills testing sheets in this Part so that you will be able to perform each skill correctly.

Remediation

Any student who does not pass both BLS skills tests will practice and undergo remediation during the remediation lesson at the end of the course.

Students who require remediation and retesting will be tested in the entire BLS skill.

BLS Skills Testing in PEARS® Course
1- and 2-Rescuer Child BLS With AED Skills Testing Sheet

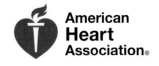

See 1- and 2-Rescuer Child BLS With AED Skills Testing Criteria and Descriptors on next page

Student Name: _____ Test Date: _____

1-Rescuer BLS and CPR Skills (circle one):	**Pass**	**Needs Remediation**	
2-Rescuer CPR Skills			
Bag-Mask (circle one):	**Pass**	**Needs Remediation**	
AED Skills (circle one):	**Pass**	**Needs Remediation**	

Skill Step	Critical Performance Criteria	✓ if done correctly	
1-Rescuer Child BLS Skills Evaluation During this first phase, evaluate the first rescuer's ability to initiate BLS and deliver high-quality CPR for 5 cycles.			
1	ASSESSES: Checks for response and for no breathing or only gasping (at least 5 seconds but no more than 10 seconds)		
2	Sends someone to ACTIVATE emergency response system		
3	Checks for PULSE (no more than 10 seconds)		
4	GIVES HIGH-QUALITY CPR:		
	• Correct compression HAND PLACEMENT	Cycle 1:	
	• ADEQUATE RATE: At least 100/min (ie, delivers each set of 30 chest compressions in 18 seconds or less), using 1 or 2 hands	Cycle 2:	Time:
	• ADEQUATE DEPTH: Delivers compressions at least one third the depth of the chest (approximately 2 inches [5 cm]) (at least 23 out of 30)	Cycle 3:	
	• ALLOWS COMPLETE CHEST RECOIL (at least 23 out of 30)	Cycle 4:	
	• MINIMIZES INTERRUPTIONS: Gives 2 breaths with pocket mask in less than 10 seconds	Cycle 5:	
Second Rescuer AED Skills Evaluation and SWITCH During this next phase, evaluate the second rescuer's ability to use the AED and both rescuers' abilities to switch roles.			
5	DURING FIFTH SET OF COMPRESSIONS: Second rescuer arrives with AED and bag-mask device, turns on AED, and applies pads		
6	First rescuer continues compressions while second rescuer turns on AED and applies pads		
7	Second rescuer clears victim, allowing AED to analyze—RESCUERS SWITCH		
8	If AED indicates a shockable rhythm, second rescuer clears victim again and delivers shock		
First Rescuer Bag-Mask Ventilation During this next phase, evaluate the first rescuer's ability to give breaths with a bag-mask device.			
9	Both rescuers RESUME HIGH-QUALITY CPR immediately after shock delivery:	Cycle 1	Cycle 2
	• SECOND RESCUER gives 15 compressions (in 9 seconds or less) immediately after shock delivery (for 2 cycles)	Time:	
	• FIRST RESCUER successfully delivers 2 breaths with bag-mask device (for 2 cycles)		
AFTER 2 CYCLES, STOP THE EVALUATION			

- If the student completes all steps successfully (a ✓ in each box to the right of Critical Performance Criteria), the student passed this scenario.
- If the student does not complete all steps successfully (as indicated by a blank box to the right of any of the Critical Performance Criteria), give the form to the student for review as part of the student's remediation.
- After reviewing the form, the student will give the form to the instructor who is reevaluating the student. The student will reperform the entire scenario, and the instructor will notate the reevaluation on this same form.
- If the reevaluation is to be done at a different time, the instructor should collect this sheet before the student leaves the classroom.

	Remediation (if needed):
Instructor Signature: _____	Instructor Signature: _____
Print Instructor Name: _____	Print Instructor Name: _____
Date: _____	Date: _____

BLS Skills Testing in PEARS® Course
1- and 2-Rescuer Child BLS With AED
Skills Testing Criteria and Descriptors

1. **Assesses victim (Steps 1 and 2, assessment and activation, must be completed within 10 seconds of arrival at scene):**
   - Checks for unresponsiveness (this MUST precede starting compressions)
   - Checks for no breathing or only gasping
2. **Sends someone to activate emergency response system (Steps 1 and 2, assessment and activation, must be completed within 10 seconds of arrival at scene):**
   - Shouts for help/directs someone to call for help AND get AED/defibrillator
3. **Checks for pulse:**
   - Checks carotid or femoral pulse
   - This should take no more than 10 seconds
4. **Delivers high-quality CPR (initiates compressions within 10 seconds of identifying cardiac arrest):**
   - Correct placement of hand(s) in center of chest
     - Child: 1 or 2 hands on lower half of breastbone
   - Compression rate of at least 100/min
     - Delivers 30 compressions in 18 seconds or less with 1 rescuer
     - Delivers 15 compressions in 9 seconds or less with 2 rescuers
   - Adequate depth for age
     - Child: at least one third the depth of the chest (approximately 2 inches [5 cm])
   - Complete chest recoil after each compression
     - Appropriate ratio for age and number of rescuers
     - 1 rescuer: 30 compressions to 2 breaths
   - Minimizes interruptions in compressions:
     - Less than 10 seconds between last compression of one cycle and first compression of next cycle
     - Compressions not interrupted until AED analyzing rhythm
     - Compressions resumed immediately after shock/no shock indicated

5-8. **Integrates prompt and proper use of AED with CPR:**
   - Turns AED on
   - Places proper-sized pads for victim's age in correct location; if available, uses child-sized pads/dose attenuator for victims younger than 8 years
   - Clears rescuers from victim for AED to analyze rhythm (pushes ANALYZE button if required by device)
   - Clears victim and delivers shock
   - Resumes chest compressions immediately after shock delivery
   - Does NOT turn off AED during CPR
   - Provides safe environment for rescuers during AED shock delivery:
     - Communicates clearly to all other rescuers to stop touching victim
     - Delivers shock to victim after all rescuers are clear of victim
   - Switches during analysis phase of AED

9. **Provides effective breaths with bag-mask device during 2-rescuer CPR:**
   - Provides effective breaths:
     - Opens airway adequately
     - Delivers each breath over 1 second
     - Delivers breaths that produce visible chest rise
     - Avoids excessive ventilation

10. **Provides high-quality chest compressions during 2-rescuer CPR:**
   - Correct placement of hand(s) in center of chest
   - Compression rate of at least 100/min
     - Delivers 15 compressions in 9 seconds or less
   - Adequate depth for age
     - Child: at least one third the depth of the chest (approximately 2 inches [5 cm])
   - Complete chest recoil after each compression
   - Appropriate ratio for age and number of rescuers
     - 2 rescuers: 15 compressions to 2 breaths
   - Minimizes interruptions in compressions
     - Less than 10 seconds between last compression of one cycle and first compression of next cycle

BLS Skills Testing in PEARS® Course
1- and 2-Rescuer Infant BLS Skills Testing Sheet

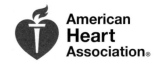

American Heart Association®

See 1- and 2-Rescuer Infant BLS Skills Testing Criteria and Descriptors on next page

Student Name: _____ Test Date: _____

1-Rescuer BLS and CPR Skills (circle one):		Pass	Needs Remediation
2-Rescuer CPR Skills			
Bag-Mask (circle one):		Pass	Needs Remediation
2 Thumb–Encircling Hands (circle one):		Pass	Needs Remediation

Skill Step	Critical Performance Criteria		✓ if done correctly
1-Rescuer Infant BLS Skills Evaluation During this first phase, evaluate the first rescuer's ability to initiate BLS and deliver high-quality CPR for 5 cycles.			
1	ASSESSES: Checks for response and for no breathing or only gasping (at least 5 seconds but no more than 10 seconds)		
2	Sends someone to ACTIVATE emergency response system (no AED available)		
3	Checks for PULSE (no more than 10 seconds)		
4	GIVES HIGH-QUALITY CPR:		
	• Correct compression FINGER PLACEMENT	Cycle 1:	
	• ADEQUATE RATE: At least 100/min (ie, delivers each set of 30 chest compressions in 18 seconds or less)	Cycle 2:	Time:
	• ADEQUATE DEPTH: Delivers compressions at least one third the depth of the chest (approximately 1½ inches [4 cm]) (at least 23 out of 30)	Cycle 3:	
	• ALLOWS COMPLETE CHEST RECOIL (at least 23 out of 30)	Cycle 4:	
	• MINIMIZES INTERRUPTIONS: Gives 2 breaths with pocket mask in less than 10 seconds	Cycle 5:	
2-Rescuer CPR and SWITCH During this next phase, evaluate the FIRST RESCUER'S ability to give breaths with a bag-mask device and give compressions by using the 2 thumb–encircling hands technique. Also evaluate both rescuers' abilities to switch roles.			
5	DURING FIFTH SET OF COMPRESSIONS: Second rescuer arrives with bag-mask device. RESCUERS SWITCH ROLES.		
6	Both rescuers RESUME HIGH-QUALITY CPR:	Cycle 1	Cycle 2
	• SECOND RESCUER gives 15 compressions in 9 seconds or less by using 2 thumb–encircling hands technique (for 2 cycles)	X	X
	• FIRST RESCUER successfully delivers 2 breaths with bag-mask device (for 2 cycles)		
AFTER 2 CYCLES, PROMPT RESCUERS TO SWITCH ROLES			
7	Both rescuers RESUME HIGH-QUALITY CPR:	Cycle 1	Cycle 2
	• FIRST RESCUER gives 15 compressions in 9 seconds or less by using 2 thumb–encircling hands technique (for 2 cycles)	Time:	Time:
	• SECOND RESCUER successfully delivers 2 breaths with bag-mask device (for 2 cycles)	X	X
AFTER 2 CYCLES, STOP THE EVALUATION			

- If the student completes all steps successfully (a ✓ in each box to the right of Critical Performance Criteria), the student passed this scenario.
- If the student does not complete all steps successfully (as indicated by a blank box to the right of any of the Critical Performance Criteria), give the form to the student for review as part of the student's remediation.
- After reviewing the form, the student will give the form to the instructor who is reevaluating the student. The student will reperform the entire scenario, and the instructor will notate the reevaluation on this same form.
- If the reevaluation is to be done at a different time, the instructor should collect this sheet before the student leaves the classroom.

	Remediation (if needed):
Instructor Signature: _____	Instructor Signature: _____
Print Instructor Name: _____	Print Instructor Name: _____
Date: _____	Date: _____

BLS Skills Testing in PEARS® Course
1- and 2-Rescuer Infant BLS
Skills Testing Criteria and Descriptors

1. **Assesses victim (Steps 1 and 2, assessment and activation, must be completed within 10 seconds of arrival at scene):**
   - Checks for unresponsiveness (this MUST precede starting compressions)
   - Checks for no breathing or only gasping

2. **Sends someone to activate emergency response system (Steps 1 and 2, assessment and activation, must be completed within 10 seconds of arrival at scene):**
   - Shouts for help/directs someone to call for help AND get AED/defibrillator
   - If alone, remains with infant to provide 2 minutes of CPR before activating emergency response system

3. **Checks for pulse:**
   - Checks brachial pulse
   - This should take no more than 10 seconds

4. **Delivers high-quality 1-rescuer CPR (initiates compressions within 10 seconds of identifying cardiac arrest):**
   - Correct placement of fingers in center of chest
     - 1 rescuer: 2 fingers just below the nipple line
   - Compression rate of at least 100/min
     - Delivers 30 compressions in 18 seconds or less
   - Adequate depth for age
     - Infant: at least one third the depth of the chest (approximately 1½ inches [4 cm])
   - Complete chest recoil after each compression
   - Appropriate ratio for age and number of rescuers
     - 1 rescuer: 30 compressions to 2 breaths
   - Minimizes interruptions in compressions:
     - Less than 10 seconds between last compression of one cycle and first compression of next cycle

5. **Switches at appropriate intervals as prompted by the instructor (for purposes of this evaluation)**

6. **Provides effective breaths with bag-mask device during 2-rescuer CPR:**
   - Provides effective breaths:
     - Opens airway adequately
     - Delivers each breath over 1 second
     - Delivers breaths that produce visible chest rise
     - Avoids excessive ventilation

7. **Provides high-quality chest compressions during 2-rescuer CPR:**
   - Correct placement of hands/fingers in center of chest
     - 2 rescuers: 2 thumb–encircling hands just below the nipple line
   - Compression rate of at least 100/min
     - Delivers 15 compressions in 9 seconds or less
   - Adequate depth for age
     - Infant: at least one third the depth of the chest (approximately 1½ inches [4 cm])
   - Complete chest recoil after each compression
   - Appropriate ratio for age and number of rescuers
     - 2 rescuers: 15 compressions to 2 breaths
   - Minimizes interruptions in compressions:
     - Less than 10 seconds between last compression of one cycle and first compression of next cycle

Part 11

Effective Team Dynamics

Effective Team Dynamics

Successful teams have medical expertise, and they master resuscitation skills. In addition, they demonstrate effective communication and team dynamics. The PEARS Provider Course stresses the importance of team roles and effective team dynamics.

The resuscitation team concept is critical to the effective stabilization of any seriously ill or injured child. As a PEARS provider you will not function as a team leader during a resuscitative effort. However, you may need to direct initial emergency care until others arrive. For example, you may be alone when you begin resuscitation. It is important that you feel prepared to start critical interventions and to direct actions of the team as they assemble until the team leader arrives. This means that you may be the team leader in the early stages when the team includes only 1 or 2 additional providers.

The single rescuer has the same priorities as a team of rescuers. Priorities include support of airway, oxygenation, ventilation, and circulation. For example, you will give oxygen to a child with low oxygen saturation or IV fluid for a child in shock. As a PEARS provider, your quick action is critical to prevent a critically ill or injured child from progressing to cardiac arrest. If the child is in cardiac arrest, immediate high-quality CPR can be lifesaving. Begin CPR as soon as you identify a child in cardiac arrest—do not wait for the resuscitation team to arrive before beginning CPR.

During the course you will have an opportunity to practice different team roles during case simulations.

Learning Objectives

After completing this Part you should be able to

- List the 8 elements of effective team dynamics
- Describe the role of each resuscitation team member
- State how teamwork affects resuscitation success

Preparation for the Course

During the course you will participate as a team member in 2 cardiac arrest case simulations. You will need to understand the roles and responsibilities of team members. These case simulations will also give you an opportunity to observe and practice the 8 elements of effective team dynamics.

Observe 8 Elements

You will watch videos of teams caring for seriously ill children. You'll be asked to identify elements of effective team dynamics.

During the case simulations, look for opportunities to practice and observe the following 8 elements of effective team dynamics (Table 1). Note examples (positive and negative) that you observe during the course.

Table 1. Eight Elements of Effective Team Dynamics

1	Closed-loop communication
2	Clear messages
3	Clear roles and responsibilities
4	Knowing your limitations
5	Knowledge sharing
6	Constructive intervention
7	Reevaluation and summarizing
8	Mutual respect

Summary of Team Roles

Roles and Responsibilities

Clear roles and responsibilities (Table 2) are critical to effective team dynamics. During the case simulations the instructor will take the role of the team leader. Each student will have the opportunity to perform different team member roles. The team leader may modify a team member's responsibilities according to his or her scope of practice.

Table 2. Summary of Team Roles and Responsibilities

Role	Responsibilities
Team leader (instructor)	In the PEARS Provider Course the instructor is the team leader in the case simulations. The instructor will provide information throughout each case, including findings from the initial impression and primary assessment.
Airway	• Open the airway by using manual maneuvers. • Suction with an appropriate device. • Give high-flow or low-flow oxygen at the appropriate flow rate. • Provide bag-mask ventilation when needed. • Evaluate the child's response to oxygen administration or airway medications.
Compressor	• Initiate chest compressions if needed. • Perform chest compressions consistent with the BLS guidelines for effective compressions. • Rotate the role of compressor with other team members about every 2 minutes during CPR. • If CPR is not needed in the case simulation, the compressor should alert the team leader that he is now available to assist with other tasks and then perform them as requested.
IV/IO/ medications	• Use a color-coded length-based resuscitation tape to estimate weight and determine equipment sizes. • Ensure patent IV/IO access. • Give a bolus of isotonic crystalloid if needed. • Evaluate response to fluid bolus. • Obtain blood tests as requested (eg, blood glucose). • Give medications as ordered by the team leader (eg, nebulized albuterol treatment).
Monitor/ defibrillator	• Place the pulse oximeter. • Attach pads/leads. • Operate the monitor/defibrillator or AED. • Safely provide electrical therapy as directed by the AED prompts.

(continued)

(continued)

Role	Responsibilities
Observer/ recorder/ timekeeper	This role may be performed by more than 1 student, based on the number of students participating in the scenario. The instructor will assign specific responsibilities so that each student is actively involved. • Help the instructor by watching the timer to make sure the simulation lasts no longer than 5 minutes. • Remind compressor to rotate with another team member about every 2 minutes during CPR. • Locate the appropriate learning station competency checklist in the Appendix to the *PEARS Provider Manual.* • Use this checklist during the case simulation to record key interventions and assessments performed by each team member. • Listen for examples of positive and negative team dynamics. • Give feedback to team members at the end of the case, based on the checklist and observation of team behaviors.

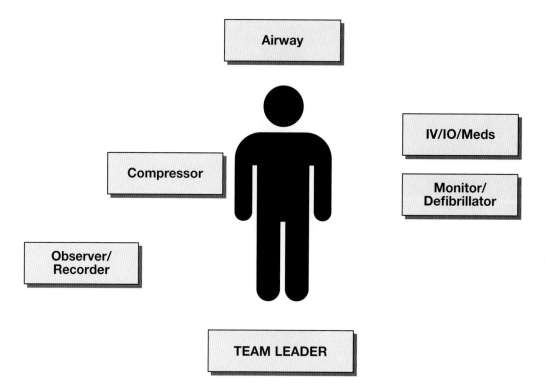

Figure 1. Suggested locations for the team leader and team members during the case simulations.

Part 12

Identification and Management of Cardiac Arrest

Overview

Pediatric cardiac arrest is uncommon. When cardiac arrest does occur, it is typically the result of progressive respiratory distress or shock. Sudden cardiac arrest resulting from a cardiac rhythm abnormality is a less common type of cardiac arrest. Prompt, high-quality CPR improves outcomes; however, the chance of survival from cardiac arrest is generally poor. In contrast, outcome from treatment of severe respiratory distress or shock in children is generally good. The focus therefore should be on prevention of cardiac arrest by

- Prevention of disease and injury that may lead to cardiac arrest
- Early recognition and management of respiratory distress and shock before the condition deteriorates to cardiac arrest

Identify and treat respiratory problems and shock before the child's condition worsens to cardiac arrest.

This Part discusses the recognition of cardiac arrest. It also discusses the importance of high-quality CPR in the treatment of cardiac arrest.

Learning Objectives

After completing this Part you should be able to

- Recall that the most common cause of cardiac arrest in children is progression of respiratory distress or shock, or both
- Identify the signs of cardiac arrest
- Describe the importance and the components of high-quality CPR in the treatment of cardiac arrest
- Recall that the heart rhythm in cardiac arrest can be shockable or nonshockable
- State the role of the AED in treatment of cardiac arrest

Preparation for the Course

During the course you will participate as part of a team in cardiac arrest case simulations. You will need to know how to identify cardiac arrest and how to perform high-quality CPR. You should also be ready to assist other team members, if needed, to make sure that high-quality CPR is performed throughout the simulated resuscitation attempt.

Definition of Cardiac Arrest

Cardiac arrest is absent or ineffective heart activity. With cardiac arrest, blood flow stops. Signs of circulation are absent. The child is unresponsive and not breathing. However, agonal gasps may be present in the first minutes after sudden cardiac arrest and should not be considered adequate breathing. There is no detectable pulse. When circulation stops, cell and organ damage begins to develop. Death may occur if immediate, high-quality CPR is not provided.

Types of Cardiac Arrest

The 2 main types of cardiac arrest are

- Hypoxic/asphyxial arrest
- Sudden cardiac arrest

Hypoxic/asphyxial arrest is the most common type of cardiac arrest in children. You may have heard the term "asphyxial" used to refer to a condition of choking or suffocation. The term *asphyxial arrest* means that the cardiac arrest is caused by an inadequate supply of oxygen to the tissues (hypoxia). This lack of oxygen can result from progression of respiratory distress, shock, or both (Figure 1).

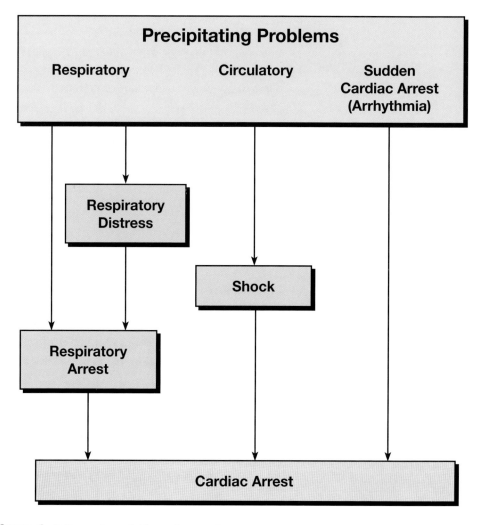

Figure 1. Pathways to pediatric cardiac arrest.

Sudden cardiac arrest is more common in adults than in children. Sudden cardiac arrest usually results from a rhythm disturbance.

Identifying a Child at Risk for Cardiac Arrest

Signs That a Child May Be at Risk for Cardiac Arrest

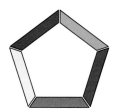

Children with the combination of severe respiratory distress and shock will likely develop cardiac arrest within minutes unless you intervene immediately. Be alert for signs of inadequate oxygenation, ventilation, and tissue perfusion (Table 1).

Table 1. Signs That a Child May Be at Risk for Cardiac Arrest

Primary Assessment	Sign
Airway	Possible upper airway obstruction
Breathing	• Slow respiratory rate or gasping • Inadequate respiratory effort • Decreased breath sounds
Circulation	• Bradycardia or decreasing heart rate • Delayed capillary refill time (typically greater than 2 seconds) • Weak central pulses • Absent peripheral pulses • Hypotension • Mottled or cyanotic skin
Disability	Decreased level of consciousness
Exposure	Cool extremities

Identification of Cardiac Arrest

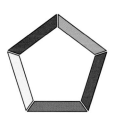

Signs of cardiac arrest are

- Unresponsiveness
- No breathing or only gasping
- No pulse (assess for no more than 10 seconds)

If a child is unresponsive and not breathing or only gasping, get help immediately and send someone to activate emergency response. Then try to palpate a central pulse (carotid or femoral) in a child or the brachial pulse in an infant. Because even healthcare providers are often unable to reliably detect a pulse, take no more than 10 seconds for a pulse check. If there is no pulse or you are not sure, start CPR, beginning with chest compressions.

Basic Life Support

BLS consists of chest compressions, airway, breathing, and defibrillation. High-quality CPR is the foundation of both basic and advanced life support. For the child in cardiac arrest, a team member should perform immediate high-quality CPR until the AED arrives. Table 2 summarizes the important components of BLS.

Table 2. Summary of Key BLS Components for Adults, Children, and Infants*

Component	Recommendations		
	Adults	**Children**	**Infants**
Recognition	Unresponsive (for all ages)		
	No breathing or no normal breathing (ie, only gasping)	No breathing or only gasping	
	No pulse palpated within 10 seconds for all ages (HCP only)		
CPR sequence	C-A-B		
Compression rate	At least 100/min		
Compression depth	At least 2 inches (5 cm)	At least ⅓ AP diameter About 2 inches (5 cm)	At least ⅓ AP diameter About 1½ inches (4 cm)
Chest wall recoil	Allow complete recoil between compressions HCPs rotate compressors every 2 minutes		
Compression interruptions	Minimize interruptions in chest compressions Attempt to limit interrruptions to <10 seconds		
Airway	Head tilt–chin lift (HCP suspected trauma: jaw thrust)		
Compression-to-ventilation ratio (until advanced airway placed)	30:2 1 or 2 rescuers	30:2 Single rescuer 15:2 2 HCP rescuers	
Ventilations: when rescuer untrained or trained and not proficient	Compressions only		
Ventilations with advanced airway (HCP)	1 breath every 6-8 seconds (8-10 breaths/min) Asynchronous with chest compressions About 1 second per breath Visible chest rise		
Defibrillation	Attach and use AED as soon as available. Minimize interruptions in chest compressions before and after shock; resume CPR beginning with compressions immediately after each shock.		

Abbreviations: AED, automated external defibrillator; AP, anterior-posterior; CPR, cardiopulmonary resuscitation; HCP, healthcare provider.
*Excluding the newly born.

High-Quality CPR

High-quality CPR is the foundation of basic and advanced life support.

Push fast	• Push at a rate of at least 100 compressions per minute.
Push hard	• Push with enough force to depress the chest at least one third the depth of the chest. This is about 1.5 inches (4 cm) in infants and 2 inches (5 cm) in children.
Allow full chest recoil	• *Release completely,* allowing the chest to fully recoil after each compression. This allows the heart to refill with blood.
Minimize interruptions	• Try to limit interruptions in chest compressions to 10 seconds or less or as needed for interventions (eg, defibrillation). Ideally, compressions are interrupted only for ventilation (until an advanced airway is placed), rhythm check, and actual shock delivery. • Once an advanced airway is in place, provide continuous chest compressions without pausing for ventilation.
Avoid excessive ventilation	• Each rescue breath should take about 1 second. • Each breath should result in visible chest rise. • After an advanced airway is in place, deliver 8 to 10 breaths/min (1 breath every 6 to 8 seconds), being careful to avoid excessive ventilation.

C-A-B Sequence

Because delays and interruptions in chest compressions reduce survival, the recommended CPR begins the sequence with chest compressions before giving rescue breaths (C-A-B rather than A-B-C). Chest compressions can be started almost immediately and require no equipment. Positioning the head and achieving a seal for mouth-to-mouth or bag-mask rescue breaths take time and may require equipment that must be assembled.

Detailed and Advanced Concepts

Hands-Only™ (chest compressions-only) CPR may be performed by untrained lay rescuers who witness the sudden collapse of an adult. However, both compressions and ventilation are important for infants and children in cardiac arrest. For an infant or child in cardiac arrest, both compressions and ventilation are recommended.

Proceed Based on the Likely Cause of Arrest

Decide what to do *first* based on the likely cause of the arrest.

If the arrest is...	Then...
Unwitnessed (assumed to be asphyxial in origin) and in out-of-hospital setting	• Shout for help. Start immediate CPR and send someone to activate emergency response and get an AED. • Perform cycles of chest compressions and ventilation for about 2 minutes. • If alone, perform cycles of chest compressions and ventilation for about 2 minutes, and then leave the victim to activate emergency response and get an AED. Return to the victim to give CPR and use the AED.
Witnessed (sudden collapse more likely to be cardiac in origin) and in in-hospital setting	• Shout for help. Send someone to activate emergency response and get an AED while you begin CPR. • If you are alone, you should activate emergency response and get an AED and then return to the victim to use the AED and give CPR. • Use the AED (and follow the voice prompts) as soon as it is available.

Pediatric BLS for Healthcare Providers Algorithm

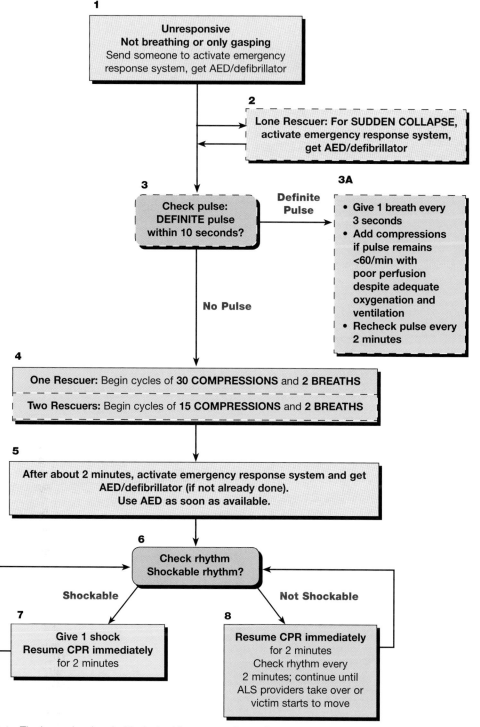

High-Quality CPR

- Rate at least 100/min
- Compression depth to at least ⅓ anterior-posterior diameter of chest, about 1½ inches (4 cm) in infants and 2 inches (5 cm) in children
- Allow complete chest recoil after each compression
- Minimize interruptions in chest compressions
- Avoid excessive ventilation

Note: The boxes bordered with dashed lines are performed by healthcare providers and not by lay rescuers

Figure 2. Pediatric BLS for Healthcare Providers Algorithm.

Shockable and Nonshockable Rhythms

The heart rhythms associated with cardiac arrest can be categorized as

- Shockable
- Nonshockable

Shockable Rhythm

A shockable rhythm is an abnormal rhythm of the heart that can be treated with CPR and an electrical shock, known as *defibrillation.* The shock may be delivered with a manual defibrillator or an automated external defibrillator (AED).

A shockable rhythm is the cause of about 5% to 15% of in-hospital and out-of-hospital cardiac arrests in children. A shockable rhythm is more likely to be present in a sudden cardiac arrest. About 27% of children with in-hospital cardiac arrest have a shockable rhythm at some point during the resuscitation. For this reason it is important to know how to give CPR and use an AED.

Nonshockable Rhythm

A nonshockable rhythm is an abnormal rhythm of the heart that is not treated with defibrillation. It is treated with CPR and medications. When possible, the cause of the arrest is treated.

Defibrillation

Only shockable rhythms are treated with defibrillation. Defibrillation does not restart the heart; it "stuns" the heart to stop the abnormal rhythm and allows the natural pacemaker cells of the heart to resume an organized rhythm. The return of an organized rhythm alone, however, does not ensure survival. The organized rhythm must ultimately produce effective pumping of the heart so that blood flow occurs. The return of blood flow is defined by the presence of palpable central pulses and is called *return of spontaneous circulation*, or *ROSC.*

It is important to provide high-quality CPR until the defibrillator is available and then immediately resume high-quality CPR after shock delivery. CPR provides blood flow until ROSC develops.

Defibrillation With an AED

Defibrillation Procedure

AEDs are available in different models. There are a few differences from model to model, but they all operate in basically the same way. The universal steps for operating an AED are the following:

Step	Action
1	**POWER ON the AED** (the AED will then guide you through the next steps). • Open the carrying case or the top of the AED. • Turn the power on (some devices will "power on" automatically when you open the lid or case).

(continued)

(continued)

Step	Action
2	**ATTACH** AED pads to the victim's bare chest. • Some AEDs are designed to be used for both children and adults. For these AEDs select the correct pad size. – *For infants:* A manual defibrillator is preferred. If a manual defibrillator is not available, use an AED equipped with a pediatric dose attenuator. If neither is available, you may use an AED without a pediatric dose attenuator. – *For children younger than 8 years:* Use child pads and a child system, if available. If child pads and a child system are not available, use an AED with adult pads and an adult system. Make sure that the adult pads do not touch each other or overlap. – *For children 8 years of age and older:* Use adult pads and an adult system (do NOT use child pads or a child system). • Peel the backing away from the AED pads. • Attach the adhesive AED pads to the victim's bare chest. Apply the pads as illustrated on the pads themselves. The typical placement* is as follows: – Place one AED pad on the victim's upper-right chest (directly below the collarbone). – Place the other pad to the side of the left nipple, with the top edge of the pad a few inches below the armpit. *For some AEDs the recommended pad placement is front and back. • Attach the AED connecting cables to the AED box (some are preconnected).
3	• "Clear" the victim and **ANALYZE** the rhythm. • If the AED prompts you, clear the victim during analysis. Be sure no one is touching the victim, not even the rescuer in charge of giving breaths. • Some AEDs will tell you to push a button to allow the AED to begin analyzing the heart rhythm; others will do that automatically. The AED may take about 5 to 15 seconds to analyze. • The AED then tells you if a shock is needed.
4	**If the AED advises a shock, it will tell you to clear the victim.** • Clear the victim before delivering the shock: be sure no one is touching the victim. • Loudly state a "clear the victim" message, such as "Everybody clear" or simply "Clear." • Look to be sure no one is in contact with the victim. • Press the **SHOCK** button. • The shock will produce a sudden contraction of the victim's muscles.
5	If no shock is needed, and after any shock delivery, **immediately resume CPR,** starting with chest compressions.
6	After 5 cycles or about 2 minutes of CPR, the AED will prompt you to repeat steps 3, 4, and 5. If "no shock advised," immediately resume CPR, beginning with chest compressions.

If 2 or more rescuers are present, 1 or more rescuers should continue CPR while 1 rescuer operates the AED.

The use of a manual defibrillator is preferred for infants in cardiac arrest. Some providers may use a manual defibrillator in AED mode, based on policies in their practice setting.

Part 13

Putting It All Together Case Discussions

Putting It All Together Case Discussions (Cases 1-6)

During the course you will watch short videos* of seriously ill or injured children with respiratory problems. Your instructor will lead the group in a discussion of the PEARS Systematic Approach for each case. These discussions will follow the format outlined below.

*To help improve your assessment skills, the PEARS Course includes videos of actual children with medical problems that you may encounter. These videos may be disturbing to some viewers. In some cases videos were looped or edited to provide you with adequate assessment time and to emphasize key teaching points.

At no time was medical care delayed for the purpose of obtaining video footage. All of these children received timely and appropriate medical care, mainly in children's hospitals. Consent was obtained before any video recording.

Initial Impression

Remember that the initial impression is your first quick (in a few seconds) "from the doorway" observation of the following:

Consciousness	Level of consciousness (eg, unresponsive, irritable, alert)
Breathing	Increased work of breathing, absent or decreased respiratory effort, or abnormal sounds heard without a stethoscope
Color	Abnormal skin color, such as pallor, mottling, or cyanosis

The purpose is to quickly identify a life-threatening problem.

Unresponsive or Responsive?

Is the child unresponsive with no breathing or only gasping? If so, provide emergency treatment and call for help.

If the child is responsive, continue the evaluate-identify-intervene sequence.

Continue the Evaluate-Identify-Intervene Sequence

Use the **evaluate-identify-intervene** sequence when caring for a seriously ill or injured child.

- *Evaluate* the child to gather information about the child's condition or status.
- *Identify* any problem by type and severity.
- *Intervene* with appropriate actions to treat the problem.

Then repeat the sequence; this process is ongoing.

Evaluate

Evaluate by using the ABCDE components of the primary assessment.

Please refer to the PEARS Systematic Approach Summary on your PEARS Pocket Reference Card or in the Appendix.

Airway

Clear	Maintainable	Not maintainable

Breathing

Respiratory Rate and Pattern	Respiratory Effort		Chest Expansion and Air Movement	Abnormal Lung and Airway Sounds		Oxygen Saturation by Pulse Oximetry
Normal	Normal	Inadequate	Normal	Stridor	Gurgling	Normal oxygen saturation (≥94%)
Irregular	Increased	• Apnea	Decreased	Snoring	Wheezing	
Fast	• Nasal flaring	• Weak cry or cough	Unequal	Barking cough	Crackles	Hypoxemia (<94%)
Slow	• Retractions		Prolonged expiration		Unequal	
Apnea	• Head bobbing			Hoarseness		
	• Seesaw respirations			Grunting		

Circulation

Heart Rate	Pulses		Capillary Refill Time	Skin Color and Temperature		Blood Pressure
	Central	Peripheral				
Normal	Normal	Normal	Normal: ≤2 seconds	Pallor	Warm skin	Normal
Fast (tachycardia)	Weak	Weak	Delayed: >2 seconds	Mottling	Cool skin	Hypotensive
Slow (bradycardia)	Absent	Absent		Cyanosis		

Disability

AVPU Pediatric Response Scale				Pupil Size; Reaction to Light		Blood Glucose	
Alert	Responds to **V**oice	Responds to **P**ain	**U**nresponsive	Normal	Abnormal	Normal	Low

Exposure

Temperature			Skin	
Normal	High	Low	Rash (eg, purpura)	Trauma (eg, injury, bleeding)

Identify by Type and Severity

Try to identify the child's problem by type and severity. Please refer to the PEARS Systematic Approach Summary on your PEARS Pocket Reference Card or in the Appendix.

Identifying Respiratory Problems		
Signs	**Type of Problem**	**Severity**

• Increased respiratory rate and effort (eg, retractions, nasal flaring)
 • Decreased air movement
 • Stridor (typically inspiratory)
 • Barking cough
 • Snoring or gurgling
 • Hoarseness
	Upper airway obstruction	**Mild respiratory distress**
		
		 • Some abnormal signs, but no signs of severe distress
		   – Increased respiratory rate
		   – Increased respiratory effort
		   – Abnormal airway and lung sounds
		   – Tachycardia
		   – Pale, cool skin
		   – Changes in level of consciousness

• Increased respiratory rate and effort (eg, retractions, nasal flaring) • Decreased air movement • Prolonged expiration • Wheezing	**Lower airway obstruction**	**Severe respiratory distress** *One or more of the following:* • Very rapid or inadequate respiratory rate
• Increased respiratory rate and effort • Decreased air movement • Grunting • Crackles	**Lung tissue disease**	• Significant or inadequate respiratory effort • Low oxygen saturation despite high-flow oxygen • Bradycardia (ominous)
• Irregular respiratory pattern • Inadequate or irregular respiratory depth and effort • Normal or decreased air movement • Possible signs of upper airway obstruction (see above)	**Disordered control of breathing**	• Cyanosis • Decreased level of consciousness

Identifying Circulatory Emergencies (Shock)		
• Tachycardia • Weak or absent peripheral pulses • Normal or weak central pulses • Delayed capillary refill time	• Changes in skin color (pallor, mottling, cyanosis) • Cool skin • Decreased level of consciousness • Decreased urine output	**Signs of poor perfusion**
Signs	**Type of Problem**	**Severity**
• Signs of poor perfusion (see above)	**Hypovolemic shock**	**Compensated shock**
• Possible signs of poor perfusion (see above) *or* • Warm, flushed skin with brisk capillary refill • Peripheral pulses may be bounding • Possible crackles • Possible petechial or purpuric rash (septic shock)	**Distributive shock**	• Signs of poor perfusion and normal systolic blood pressure **Hypotensive shock** • Signs of poor perfusion and low systolic blood pressure (hypotension)

Part 9

Intervene

For a quick reference on management of respiratory and circulatory problems, see the Management of Respiratory Emergencies and Management of Shock Flowcharts on your PEARS Pocket Reference Card or in the Appendix.

Case 1 Notes

_____

_____

_____

Case 2 Notes

_____

_____

_____

Case 3 Notes

_____

_____

_____

Case 4 Notes

_____

_____

_____

_____

Case 5 Notes

_____

_____

_____

_____

Case 6 Notes

_____

_____

_____

_____

Appendix

Appendix Contents

Learning Aids

The Appendix contains learning aids that you will use during core case discussions. Also, the observer/recorder team members will use the learning station competency checklists to record the performance of the team during the cardiac arrest case simulations.

Core Case Discussions

PEARS Systematic Approach Algorithm

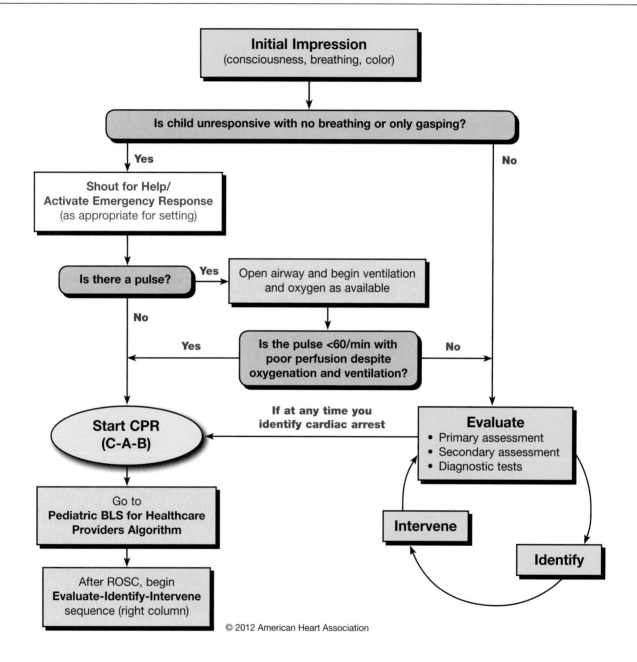

Initial Impression
(consciousness, breathing, color)

Is child unresponsive with no breathing or only gasping?

Yes

**Shout for Help/
Activate Emergency Response**
(as appropriate for setting)

No

Is there a pulse?

Yes

Open airway and begin ventilation
and oxygen as available

No

**Is the pulse <60/min with
poor perfusion despite
oxygenation and ventilation?**

Yes

No

**Start CPR
(C-A-B)**

If at any time you
identify cardiac arrest

Evaluate
• Primary assessment
• Secondary assessment
• Diagnostic tests

Go to
**Pediatric BLS for Healthcare
Providers Algorithm**

Intervene

Identify

After ROSC, begin
Evaluate-Identify-Intervene
sequence (right column)

© 2012 American Heart Association

PEARS Systematic Approach Summary

Initial Impression	Your first quick *(in a few seconds)* "from the doorway" observation

Consciousness	Level of consciousness (eg, unresponsive, irritable, alert)
Breathing	Increased work of breathing, absent or decreased respiratory effort, or abnormal sounds heard without auscultation
Color	Abnormal skin color, such as pallor, mottling, or cyanosis
	The purpose is to quickly identify a life-threatening problem.

Is the child unresponsive with no breathing or only gasping?

If YES:

- Shout for help.
- Activate emergency response as appropriate for setting.
- Check for a pulse.
- Begin lifesaving interventions as needed.

If NO:

- Continue the evaluate-identify-intervene sequence.

Use the ***evaluate-identify-intervene*** sequence when caring for a seriously ill or injured child.

- *Evaluate* the child to gather information about the child's condition or status.
- *Identify* any problem by type and severity.
- *Intervene* with appropriate actions to treat the problem.

Then repeat the sequence; this process is ongoing.

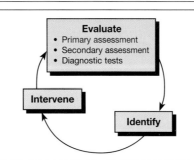

If at any time you identify a life-threatening problem, immediately begin appropriate interventions. Activate emergency response as indicated in your practice setting.

Evaluate	*"Evaluate" consists of the primary assessment (ABCDE), secondary assessment, and diagnostic tests.*

Primary Assessment	A rapid, hands-on ABCDE approach to evaluate respiratory, cardiac, and neurologic function; this step includes assessment of vital signs and pulse oximetry

Airway

Clear	Maintainable	Not maintainable

Breathing

Respiratory Rate and Pattern	Respiratory Effort		Chest Expansion and Air Movement	Abnormal Lung and Airway Sounds		Oxygen Saturation by Pulse Oximetry

Normal
Irregular
Fast
Slow
Apnea
	Normal
	Increased
	• Nasal flaring
	• Retractions
	• Head bobbing
	• Seesaw
	  respirations
		Inadequate
		• Apnea
		• Weak cry or
		  cough
			Normal
			Decreased
			Unequal
			Prolonged expiration
				Stridor
				Snoring
				Barking cough
				Hoarseness
				Grunting
					Gurgling
					Wheezing
					Crackles
					Unequal
						Normal oxygen
						  saturation (≥94%)
						Hypoxemia (<94%)

Circulation

Heart Rate	Pulses		Capillary Refill Time	Skin Color and Temperature		Blood Pressure
Normal Fast (tachycardia) Slow (bradycardia)	***Central*** Normal Weak Absent	***Peripheral*** Normal Weak Absent	Normal: ≤2 seconds Delayed: >2 seconds	Pallor Mottling Cyanosis	Warm skin Cool skin	Normal Hypotensive

Disability

AVPU Pediatric Response Scale				Pupil Size: Reaction to Light		Blood Glucose	
Alert	Responds to **V**oice	Responds to **P**ain	**U**nresponsive	Normal	Abnormal	Normal	Low

Exposure

Temperature			Skin	
Normal	High	Low	Rash (eg, purpura)	Trauma (eg, injury, bleeding)

Secondary Assessment	A focused medical history and a focused physical exam

Diagnostic Tests	Laboratory, radiographic, and other advanced tests that help to identify the child's condition and diagnosis

Identify	*Identify the child's problem as respiratory, circulatory, or both. Determine the type and severity of the problem(s). The table below lists common clinical signs that typically correlate with a specific type of problem and its severity.*

	Type	Severity
Respiratory	• Upper airway obstruction • Lower airway obstruction • Lung tissue disease • Disordered control of breathing	• Mild respiratory distress • Severe respiratory distress
Circulatory	• Hypovolemic shock • Distributive (eg, septic, anaphylactic) shock • Obstructive shock • Cardiogenic shock	• Compensated shock • Hypotensive shock
Cardiac Arrest		

Identifying Respiratory Problems

Signs	Type of Problem	Severity

• Increased respiratory rate and effort (eg, retractions, nasal flaring)
• Decreased air movement
• Stridor (typically inspiratory)
• Barking cough
• Snoring or gurgling
• Hoarseness
	Upper airway obstruction	**Mild respiratory distress**
		• Some abnormal signs, but no signs of severe distress
		  – Increased respiratory rate
		  – Increased respiratory effort
		  – Abnormal airway and lung sounds
		  – Tachycardia
		  – Pale, cool skin
		  – Changes in level of consciousness

• Increased respiratory rate and effort (eg, retractions, nasal flaring) • Decreased air movement • Prolonged expiration • Wheezing	**Lower airway obstruction**	**Severe respiratory distress** *One or more of the following:* • Very rapid or inadequate respiratory rate • Significant or inadequate respiratory effort • Low oxygen saturation despite high-flow oxygen • Bradycardia (ominous) • Cyanosis • Decreased level of consciousness
• Increased respiratory rate and effort • Decreased air movement • Grunting • Crackles	**Lung tissue disease**	
• Irregular respiratory pattern • Inadequate or irregular respiratory depth and effort • Normal or decreased air movement • Possible signs of upper airway obstruction (see above)	**Disordered control of breathing**	

Identifying Circulatory Emergencies (Shock)

• Tachycardia • Weak or absent peripheral pulses • Normal or weak central pulses • Delayed capillary refill time	• Changes in skin color (pallor, mottling, cyanosis) • Cool skin • Decreased level of consciousness • Decreased urine output	**Signs of poor perfusion**
Signs	**Type of Problem**	**Severity**
• Signs of poor perfusion (see above)	**Hypovolemic shock**	**Compensated shock** • Signs of poor perfusion and normal systolic blood pressure
• Possible signs of poor perfusion (see above) *or* • Warm, flushed skin with brisk capillary refill • Peripheral pulses may be bounding • Possible crackles • Possible petechial or purpuric rash (septic shock)	**Distributive shock**	**Hypotensive shock** • Signs of poor perfusion and low systolic blood pressure (hypotension)

Intervene	*On the basis of your identification of the problem, intervene with appropriate actions. Your actions will be determined by your scope of practice and local protocol.*

Table 1. Normal Respiratory Rates by Age

Age	Breaths/min
Infant (younger than 1 year)	30 to 60
Toddler (1 to 3 years)	24 to 40
Preschooler (4 to 5 years)	22 to 34
School-age child (6 to 12 years)	18 to 30
Adolescent (13 to 18 years)	12 to 16

Reproduced from Hazinski MF. Children are different. In: Hazinski MF. *Manual of Pediatric Critical Care*. St Louis, MO: Mosby; 1999:1-13, copyright Elsevier. From Hazinski MF. Children are different. In: Hazinski MF. *Nursing Care of the Critically Ill Child*. 2nd ed. St Louis, MO: Mosby-Year Book; 1992:1-17, copyright Elsevier.

Table 2. Normal Heart Rates (per Minute) by Age

Age	Awake Rate	Mean	Sleeping Rate
Newborn to 3 months	85 to 205	140	80 to 160
3 months to 2 years	100 to 190	130	75 to 160
2 years to 10 years	60 to 140	80	60 to 90
Older than 10 years	60 to 100	75	50 to 90

Modified from Gillette PC, Garson A Jr, Crawford F, Ross B, Ziegler V, Buckles D. Dysrhythmias. In: Adams FH, Emmanouilides GC, Reimenschneider TA, eds. *Moss' Heart Disease in Infants, Children, and Adolescents*. 4th ed. Baltimore, MD: Williams & Wilkins; 1989:925-939.

Table 3. Normal Blood Pressures by Age

Age	Systolic Blood Pressure (mm Hg)		Diastolic Blood Pressure (mm Hg)	
	Female	Male	Female	Male
Neonate (1 day)	60 to 76	60 to 74	31 to 45	30 to 44
Neonate (4 days)	67 to 83	68 to 84	37 to 53	35 to 53
Infant (1 month)	73 to 91	74 to 94	36 to 56	37 to 55
Infant (3 months)	78 to 100	81 to 103	44 to 64	45 to 65
Infant (6 months)	82 to 102	87 to 105	46 to 66	48 to 68
Infant (1 year)	86 to 104	85 to 103	40 to 58	37 to 56
Child (2 years)	88 to 105	88 to 106	45 to 63	42 to 61
Child (7 years)	96 to 113	97 to 115	57 to 75	57 to 76
Adolescent (15 years)	110 to 127	113 to 131	65 to 83	64 to 83

This table summarizes the range of systolic and diastolic blood pressures according to age and gender from 1 standard deviation below to 1 standard deviation above the mean in the first year of life and from the 50th to 95th percentile (assuming the 50th percentile for height) for children 1 year of age or older.

Blood pressure ranges for neonate and infant (1 to 6 months) are from Gemelli M, Manganaro R, Mamì C, De Luca F. Longitudinal study of blood pressure during the 1st year of life. *Eur J Pediatr.* 1990;149:318-320.

Blood pressure ranges for infant (1 year), child, and adolescent are from National High Blood Pressure Education Program Working Group on High Blood Pressure in Children and Adolescents. *The Fourth Report on the Diagnosis, Evaluation, and Treatment of High Blood Pressure in Children and Adolescents.* Bethesda, MD: National Heart, Lung, and Blood Institute; 2005. NIH publication 05-5267.

Table 4. Threshold by Age of Systolic Blood Pressure Indicating Hypotension

Age	Systolic Blood Pressure
Term neonates (0 to 28 days)	Less than 60 mm Hg
Infants (1 to 12 months)	Less than 70 mm Hg
Children 1 to 10 years (5th blood pressure percentile)	Less than 70 + (age in years × 2) mm Hg
Children older than 10 years	Less than 90 mm Hg

Table 5. Consensus Definition of Hypoglycemia

Age	Consensus Definition of Hypoglycemia
Preterm neonates **Term neonates**	Less than 45 mg/dL
Infants **Children** **Adolescents**	Less than 60 mg/dL

Table 6. Oxygen Saturation Readings

Oxygen Saturation Reading	Intervention
94% or higher when breathing room air	Oxygenation is adequate; validate by clinical assessment
Less than 94% (hypoxemia) when breathing room air	Give supplementary oxygen
Less than 90% with supplementary oxygen (severe hypoxemia)	Get help; additional interventions are usually required, including bag-mask ventilation when level of consciousness is decreased

General Management for All Patients
• Get help
• Support airway (positioning, suctioning, manual maneuvers, OPA)
• Assist ventilation if needed
• Give oxygen
• Monitor respiratory rate and effort, oxygen saturation by pulse oximetry, heart rate, level of consciousness
• Ensure vascular access as needed
• Perform frequent reassessments

Upper Airway Obstruction		
Specific Management for Selected Conditions		
Croup	**Anaphylaxis**	**Foreign-Body Airway Obstruction (FBAO)**
• Nebulized epinephrine • Consider corticosteroids	• Epinephrine by autoinjector • Nebulized albuterol (or MDI) PRN • 20 mL/kg NS/LR bolus PRN for hypotension	• Follow steps for relief of FBAO • Remove foreign body if seen

Lower Airway Obstruction	
Specific Management for Selected Conditions	
Bronchiolitis	**Asthma**
• Consider nebulized epinephrine or albuterol	• Nebulized albuterol (or MDI) • Consider corticosteroids

Lung Tissue Disease
Specific Management for Infectious Pneumonia
Pneumonia
• Give first dose of antibiotic (for infectious pneumonia) • Nebulized albuterol (or MDI) PRN • Treat fever

Disordered Control of Breathing		
Specific Management for Selected Conditions		
Increased ICP	**Poisoning/Overdose**	**Neuromuscular Disease**
• Elevate head of bed; keep patient's head in midline • Treat fever • Assist ventilation	• Assist ventilation • Contact poison control	• Assist ventilation • Suction as needed

Management of Shock Flowchart

General Management for All Patients
• Get help
• Position the child
• Give high-flow oxygen
• Support airway and ventilation as needed
• Ensure vascular (IV/IO) access
• Begin IV/IO fluid bolus therapy for shock
• Monitor oxygen saturation, heart rate, peripheral pulses, capillary refill, skin color and temperature, blood pressure, urine output, level of consciousness, blood glucose
• Perform frequent reassessments
Hypovolemic Shock
• 20 mL/kg NS/LR bolus (repeat as needed)
• Control external bleeding (if present)
Distributive (eg, Septic) Shock
• 20 mL/kg NS/LR bolus (repeat as needed)

Respiratory Skills Practice Checklist

Based on students' scope of practice, the PEARS Course may include hands-on practice with some of the following respiratory management skills:

Skill	✓ if done correctly
Opening the airway	
Opens airway by using head tilt–chin lift maneuver while keeping mouth open in the unconscious child (jaw thrust for trauma victim)	
Suctioning	
Demonstrates appropriate use of suction device to remove copious or thick secretions	
Oxygen delivery devices	
Ask student: *"What device delivers high-flow oxygen, and what is the correct flow rate?"*	
Verbalizes correct flow rates for the following high-flow oxygen device: • Nonrebreathing mask: 10 to 15 L/min	

(continued)

(continued)

Skill	✓ if done correctly
Ask student: *"What devices deliver low-flow oxygen, and what are the correct flow rates?"*	
Verbalizes correct flow rates for the following low-flow devices: • Nasal cannula: 0.25 to 4 L/min • Simple oxygen mask: 6 to 10 L/min	
OPA	
Ask student: *"When is the OPA used?"*	
States that OPA is used only in the unconscious child without a gag reflex	
Selects correctly sized airway	
Inserts OPA correctly	
Evaluates breathing after insertion of OPA	
Gives 2 breaths (1 second each) with bag-mask	
Suctions with OPA in place; states suctioning not to exceed 10 seconds	
Bag-mask device	
Opens airway, uses E-C clamp technique, gives breaths with bag-mask device, causing observable chest rise. Gives 1 breath every 3 to 5 seconds for 30 seconds.	
Respiratory physical exam	
Demonstrates auscultation points for respiratory physical exam	
Nebulizer	
Identifies components of nebulizer equipment; verbalizes correct oxygen flow rate; verbalizes correct technique for administering medication	
Prepares equipment for delivering medication by nebulizer	
MDI	
Verbalizes or demonstrates correct technique for administering medication via MDI	

Circulatory Skills Practice Checklist

Based on students' scope of practice, the PEARS Course may include hands-on practice with some of the following circulatory management skills:

Skill	✓ if done correctly
Monitor/AED	
Applies ECG leads correctly: • White lead: to right shoulder • Red lead: to left ribs, flank • Black, green, or brown lead: to left shoulder	
Demonstrates correct operation of monitor: • Turns monitor on • Selects appropriate lead setting (lead II) • Adjusts ECG size and volume • Prints a rhythm strip	
Selects correct defibrillation pads for infant or child; places pads in correct position	
Demonstrates safe and correct defibrillation with an AED or manual defibrillator in AED mode	
Vascular access	
Ask student: *"What is the next action for a child with poor circulation?"*	
Verbalizes that child needs urgent vascular access; calls for help	
Verbalizes that isotonic crystalloid boluses should be used in shock	
States appropriate type of fluid to give as a rapid infusion	
Optional, based on scope of practice: **IV/IO bolus**	
Practices giving an IV/IO bolus with syringe and 3-way stopcock	
Demonstrates correct use of equipment to give bolus	
Positioning the shock patient	
Demonstrates correct positioning of a child in hypovolemic or distributive shock: lying on the back, faceup, with head lowered so that the feet are raised above the heart.	
Epinephrine autoinjector	
Discusses correct technique for administering medication via an epinephrine autoinjector	

Learning Station Competency Checklists

Cardiac Arrest: Shockable Rhythm Team Dynamics Practice	The observer/recorder should use this checklist during case simulations to check off the performance of team members and provide feedback.

Critical Performance Steps
Each Team Member
___ Demonstrates effective team dynamics (see "Effective Team Dynamics" below)
Team Member Role: Airway
___ Performs manual maneuvers to open airway*
___ Simulates suctioning of airway*
___ Initiates assisted ventilation with bag-mask device attached to (simulated) high-flow oxygen
___ Performs effective ventilation with bag-mask device
___ Evaluates response to oxygen administration or airway medications
Team Member Role: Compressor
___ Begins initial steps of CPR
___ Activates emergency response (or sends someone to do so)
___ Identifies cardiac arrest
___ Performs high-quality chest compressions consistent with BLS Guidelines
___ Rotates role of compressor with other team members about every 2 minutes during CPR
Team Member Role: IV/IO/Medications
___ Simulates placement of vascular access (IV/IO)*
___ Uses color-coded length-based resuscitation tape to estimate weight and determine equipment sizes
___ Gives medications as ordered by team leader
Team Member Role: Monitor/Defibrillator
___ Turns on AED
___ Attaches pads/leads in correct positions
___ Operates monitor/defibrillator or AED as needed
___ Safely provides electrical therapy as directed by AED prompts

*If indicated and within student's scope of practice.

Effective Team Dynamics	
Closed-loop communication	Knowledge sharing
Clear messages	Constructive intervention
Clear roles and responsibilities	Reevaluation and summarizing
Knowing one's limitations	Mutual respect

Cardiac Arrest: Nonshockable Rhythm Team Dynamics Practice	*The observer/recorder should use this checklist during case simulations to check off the performance of team members and provide feedback.*

Critical Performance Steps
Each Team Member
___ Demonstrates effective team dynamics (see "Effective Team Dynamics" below)
Team Member Role: Airway
___ Performs manual maneuvers to open airway*
___ Simulates suctioning of airway*
___ Initiates assisted ventilation with bag-mask device attached to (simulated) high-flow oxygen
___ Performs effective ventilation with bag-mask device
___ Evaluates response to oxygen administration or airway medications
Team Member Role: Compressor
___ Begins initial steps of CPR
___ Activates emergency response (or sends someone to do so)
___ Identifies cardiac arrest
___ Performs high-quality chest compressions consistent with BLS Guidelines
___ Rotates role of compressor with other team members about every 2 minutes during CPR
Team Member Role: IV/IO/Medications
___ Simulates placement of vascular access (IV/IO)*
___ Uses color-coded length-based resuscitation tape to estimate weight and determine equipment sizes
___ Gives medications as ordered by team leader
Team Member Role: Monitor/Defibrillator
___ Turns on AED
___ Attaches pads/leads in correct position
___ Operates monitor/defibrillator or AED as needed
___ Safely provides electrical therapy as directed by AED prompts

*If indicated and within student's scope of practice.

Effective Team Dynamics	
Closed-loop communication	Knowledge sharing
Clear messages	Constructive intervention
Clear roles and responsibilities	Reevaluation and summarizing
Knowing one's limitations	Mutual respect

Index

Index

Additional Training Options From the American Heart Association

To advance your emergency cardiovascular care knowledge and skills, the American Heart Association has also developed these courses.

To enhance or specialize your training, consider these courses:

Pediatric Advanced Life Support (PALS) uses a scenario-based, team approach to teach emergency management and treatment of pediatric respiratory and cardiac arrest. The course is available as classroom-based or as eLearning, which offers continuing education credit.

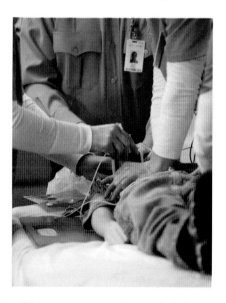

To learn more or purchase this course, contact your Training Center or visit **www.heart.org/cpr**.

Learn:® Rhythm Pediatric introduces students to normal pediatric cardiac rhythms and prepares students to recognize basic pediatric cardiac arrhythmias in clinical practice. This online course features a combination of audio, animation, interactive activities, self-assessment portions, and debriefing with suggestions for improvement.

To learn about continuing education credit or purchase this course, contact your Training Center or visit **www.OnlineAHA.org**.

Looking for a basic life support (BLS) course? AHA offers classroom training:

The **BLS for Healthcare Providers Classroom Course** is designed to provide a wide variety of healthcare professionals the ability to recognize several life-threatening emergencies, provide CPR, use an AED, and relieve choking in a safe, timely, and effective manner.

To learn more or purchase this course, contact your Training Center or visit **www.heart.org/cpr**.

For your BLS renewal training, try these online courses:

In **BLS for Healthcare Providers Online Part 1,** students work through case-based scenarios and get feedback as they move through critical checkpoints.

HeartCode® BLS Part 1 uses eSimulation technology so students "virtually treat" sudden cardiac arrest patients and follow interactive, simulated cases for feedback and debriefing.

Part 1 of each course requires 1 to 2 hours to complete, plus additional time for a hands-on skills session.

To learn more or purchase these courses, contact your training center or visit **www.OnlineAHA.org**.

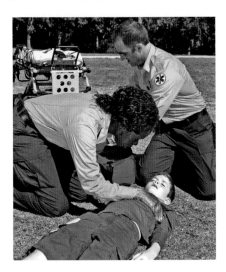

Healthcare Programs From the American Heart Association

The American Heart Association has created a variety of programs and products for the public, healthcare professionals, and legislators that educate and raise awareness about cardiovascular health and disease prevention. Many also provide tools and information to help individuals and groups make an impact on improving survival in their communities. Learn more and get involved today.

Get With The Guidelines®

This suite of quality-improvement products empowers hospital teams to deliver heart and stroke care consistent with the most up-to-date scientific guidelines.

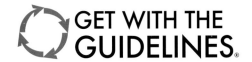

To learn more, visit **www.heart.org/resuscitation**.

Mission: Lifeline®

This national initiative seeks to improve the overall quality of care for ST-segment elevation myocardial infarction (STEMI) patients by improving systems of care.

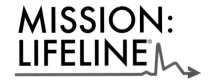

Learn more at **www.heart.org/missionlifeline**.